BRIDGING THE FAMILY-PROFESSIONAL GAP

ABOUT THE EDITORS

Dr. Billy T. Ogletree received the Certificate of Clinical Competence from the American Speech-Language-Hearing Association in 1982 and has practiced professionally as a speech-language pathologist since that time. His professional career has included interdisciplinary team-based experience in a day development center, an intermediate care facility for persons with mental retardation, three university speech and hearing clinics, and a university affiliated program (UAP).

Dr. Ogletree earned his Ph.D. in Speech-Language Pathology from Florida State University in 1988 and is currently an associate professor in the Communication Disorders Program at Western Carolina University. Dr. Ogletree has published/presented in the fields of interdisciplinary practice, developmental disabilities, early intervention, and communication disorders

Dr. Martin A. Fischer received the Certificate of Clinical Competence from the American Speech-Language-Hearing Association in 1980. His professional career has included interdisciplinary team-based experiences in four public school districts, two university speech and hearing clinics, and a major medical center.

Dr. Fischer earned his Ph.D. in Speech-Language Pathology from the University of Oregon in 1983 and is currently an associate professor in the Communication Disorders Program at Western Carolina University. Dr. Fischer has published/presented in the fields of developmental disabilities, technology, early intervention, and communication disorders.

Dr. Jane B. Schulz received her Ed.D. in Special Education from Auburn University in 1971. Her professional career has included team-based experiences in numerous public school and university settings. Currently, Dr. Schulz is a professor emerita in the Special Education Program at Western Carolina University. Dr. Schulz has published/presented extensively with primary emphases upon mainstreaming and a parent issues. Her co-authored 1995 book entitled *Mainstreaming Exceptional Students: A Guide for Classroom Teachers* (4th ed.) is considered a landmark text in special education.

BRIDGING THE FAMILY-PROFESSIONAL GAP

Facilitating Interdisciplinary Services for Children with Disabilities

Edited by

BILLY T. OGLETREE, Ph.D.

MARTIN A. FISCHER, Ph.D

JANE B. SCHULZ, Ed.D.

Western Carolina University

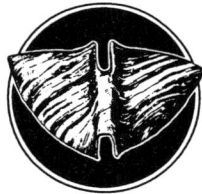

Charles C Thomas
PUBLISHER • LTD.
SPRINGFIELD • ILLINOIS • U.S.A.

Published and Distributed Throughout the World by

CHARLES C THOMAS • PUBLISHER, LTD.
2600 South First Street
Springfield, Illinois 62794-9265

ISBN 0-398-06988-3 (cloth)
ISBN 0-398-06989-1 (paper)

Library of Congress Catalog Card Number: 99-23602

With THOMAS BOOKS *careful attention is given to all details of manufacturing
and design. It is the Publisher's desire to present books that are satisfactory as to their
physical qualities and artistic possibilities and appropriate for their particular use.*
THOMAS BOOKS *will be true to those laws of quality that assure a good name
and good will.*

Printed in the United States of America
CR-R-3

Library of Congress Cataloging-in-Publication Data

Bridging the family-professional gap : facilitating interdisciplinary
services for children with disabilities / edited by Billy T. Ogletree,
Martin A. Fischer, and Jane B. Schulz.
    p.   cm.
  Includes bibliographical references and index.
   ISBN 0-398-06988-3 (cloth). -- ISBN 0-398-06989-1 (paper)
   1. Handicapped children--Services for--United States. 2. Parents
of handicapped children--Services for--United States. I. Ogletree,
Billy T. II. Fischer, Martin A. (Martin Alan), 1950-
III. Schulz, Jane B., 1924-
HV888.5.B74 1999
362.4'048'0830973--dc21   99-23602
                                                         CIP

This book is dedicated to the memory of Alan Johnson.
His influence with the children and families of Jackson County,
North Carolina is missed.

CONTRIBUTORS

W. DALE BROTHERTON, PH.D.
Associate Professor
Counseling Program
Western Carolina University
Cullowhee, North Carolina

KATHLEEN M. CARR, MSW, LCSW
Clinical Social Worker
Raytown Consolidated School District No. 2
Raytown, Missouri

STEVEN COLSON, PH.D.
Educational Diagnostician
Department of Special Education
The University of Kansas Medical Center
Kansas City, Kansas

DEBORA B. DANIELS, M.A., CCC-SLP
Coordinator of Speech Pathology
Child Development Unit
The University of Kansas Medical Center
Kansas City, Kansas

MARY DECK, PH.D.
Professor
Counseling Program
Western Carolina University
Cullowhee, North Carolina

KEVIN L. DEWEAVER, PH.D.
Professor
School of Social work
University of Georgia
Athens, Georgia

WINNIE DUNN, PH.D., OTR FOTA
Professor and Chair
Occupational Therapy Education
The University of Kansas Medical Center
Kansas City, Kansas

BLAIR M. EIG, M.D.
President, Medical Staff
Children's National Medical Center
Associate Clinical Professor
George Washington University School of Medicine
Washington, DC

MARTIN A. FISCHER, PH.D., CCC-SLP
Associate Professor
Communication Disorders Program
Western Carolina University
Cullowhee, North Carolina

CAROLYN GRAFF, RNC, MN
Director of ISEE (Sibling) Project
School of Nursing
The University of Kansas Medical Center
Kansas City, Kansas

SANDY KEENER, M.A., CCC-AP
Audiologist
Child Development Unit
The University of Kansas Medical Center
Kansas City, Kansas

NANCY P. KROPF, PH.D.
Associate Dean
School of Social Work
The University of Georgia
Athens, Georgia

SARAH MCCAMMAN, MS, RD, LD
Director of Training in Nutrition
Child Development Unit
The University of Kansas Medical Center
Kansas City, Kansas

BETH DALTON MOFFITT. M.A., CCC-SLP
Speech-Language Pathologist
Diamond Lake School District #76
Mundelein, Illinois

BILLY T. OGLETREE, PH.D., CCC-SLP
Associate Professor
Communication Disorders Program
Western Carolina University
Cullowhee, North Carolina

THOMAS OREN, PH.D.
Assistant Professor
Special Education Program
Western Carolina University
Cullowhee, North Carolina

FRANCES PALMER, M.S.
Certified School Counselor
Chapel Hill Independent School District
Tyler, Texas

MATTHEW REESE, PH.D.
Psychologist
Child Development Unit
The University of Kansas Medical Center
Kansas City, Kansas

JANE RUES, ED.D., OTR, FAOTA
Professor and Chair
Occupational Therapy Education Program
Rockhurst University
Kansas City, Missouri

JANE B. SCHULZ, ED.D.
Professor Emerita
Special Education Program
Western Carolina University
Cullowhee, North Carolina

SONYA VELLET, PH.D.
Psychologist
Child Development Unit
The University of Kansas Medical Center
Kansas City, Kansas

KATHERINE LeGUIN WHITE, PH.D.
Head, Department of Physical Therapy
Western Carolina University
Cullowhee, North Carolina

PREFACE

The gap between families of children with disabilities and the allied health, educational, and medical community is real. Its size fluctuates, dependent in large part upon the caring nature of service providers. As professionals communicate effectively, demonstrate sensitivity, and exhibit empathy, the gap narrows. These types of behaviors can be referred to as professional caring.

Unfortunately, professionals' efforts to be caring can get lost in the maze of service delivery. Deadlines, cost efficiency, and professional distancing, among other things, may result in fragmented, impersonal care. This, in turn, often leads to a broader gap between families and professionals.

This book is a specific effort to bridge the family-professional gap. Its premises are simple. First, ideal care is provided through team models that include family members in decision-making and service delivery circles. Second, some families enter these circles at a disadvantage due to their lack of knowledge of family roles within discipline/team-specific practices. Third, due to this disadvantage, many families may not take active roles in care or may simply get lost in the service provision process.

What follows is a reader-friendly introduction to team-based service delivery. Although a variety of team models are introduced, interdisciplinary teams are highlighted due to their broad acceptance. Aside from an introduction to teaming, this book consists of a chapter specific to family issues and chapters written by practicing representatives of thirteen allied health, educational, or medical disciplines. Each of the thirteen discipline-specific chapters provides an overview of the roles and responsibilities of discipline members, the discipline's contributions to interdisciplinary practice, and families' roles in optimal service delivery. Chapters also include family questions obtained via a national survey of families of children with disabilities. These questions are answered by chapter authors, and frequently responses are also included from the third editor, a parent who has a child with disabilities and is a special educator. Finally, each chapter includes a case example where chapter points are illustrated within real world scenarios.

As editors, we believe that this book has a place on most bookshelves. It is not only an excellent guide to services for families, it represents something unusual in that family voices are provided a forum for expression. Hearing and learning from these voices is the first step to bridging the family-professional gap.

Billy T. Ogletree
Martin A. Fischer
Jane B. Schulz

ACKNOWLEDGMENTS

The editors are deeply grateful to the families and professionals who contributed to the contents of this book. Their comments, questions, and insights will provide immeasurable benefits to the reader. We would also like to express our gratitude to the many individuals who assisted with the collection and organization of survey data. Two former graduate students at Western Carolina University, Laura Jenkins and Jennifer Munn, deserve special mention. Finally, this book would not have been possible without the tireless efforts of Judy Revere, whose cheerful and competent manuscript preparation made us know that there was light at the end of the tunnel.

CONTENTS

BRIDGING THE FAMILY-PROFESSIONAL GAP

Chapter 1

INTRODUCTION TO TEAMING

BILLY T. OGLETREE

The purpose of this chapter is straightforward—to provide an introduction to teaming that facilitates effective service delivery for families and beginning professionals. The chapter includes an overview of teaming and basic team models, a review of characteristics of optimal interdisciplinary team functioning, and a discussion of families as team members. It concludes with suggestions for family members and professionals beginning the team process together.

TEAMS AND SERVICE DELIVERY FOR CHILDREN
WITH DISABILITIES

Prior to discussing specific team models, it is useful to define what a team is and briefly discuss the history of team-based service delivery for children with disabilities. Most dictionaries define *team* with words like "group" or "collective" and describe team processes as "collaborative." For the purposes of this text, a team will be considered a group of two or more persons who work together from equal standing to facilitate positive outcomes for children and families. This definition has three components. First, to be a team two or more persons must work together in the provision of care. Second, to be a team, members must function as equals in decision-making. Finally, teams must have goals that identify and promote the welfare of children and families.

Teams have been a part of service provision to children for some time. Ackerly (1947) noted that teams were present in care as early as the 1920s. By the mid to latter part of this century, a team approach became broadly recognized as preferred practice for children with developmental disabilties (Allen, Holm, & Schiefelbusch, 1978; Beck, 1962; Hart, 1977). Golin and

Ducanis (1981) identified holistic interventions and legislative mandates as two factors significant in the rise of team-based service delivery. According to these authors, efforts to view children as wholes rather than parts provided an impetus for professionals to function in teams. Likewise, federal legislation such as Public Laws 94-142 (IDEA) and 99-457 strongly supported team-based service delivery. With the rise of team practice, various models of team functioning emerged that mirrored best practice trends.

Team Models

There are three widely accepted models for team practice. Multidisciplinary teams have the longest history and most closely parallel the medical model of service delivery. According to Rokusek (1995), the multidisciplinary team has a leader who is ultimately responsible for decision-making specific to team actions. She also notes that multidisciplinary teams may consist of members who have unequal roles in team processes. (The reader should note that this is not consistent with the definition of teams promoted in this text.) Finally, Rokusek (1995) noted that with multidisciplinary teams "the focus is not on the interdependent working relationship of the team members, but rather on the input of the team members to the team leader, who assimilates and directs final outcomes/recommendations" (p. 5).

An extreme contrast to the multidisciplinary model is the transdisciplinary team. The transdisciplinary team represents the newest team structure and has gained popularity with professionals serving infants, toddlers, and their families (see Chapter 11). Lyon and Lyon (1980) described three characteristics of the transdisciplinary team. First, there is joint service delivery. This simply refers to the fact that transdisciplinary teams perform services as a collective unit. Second, there is an interdependence in training. That is, members of the transdisciplinary team take responsibility to train each other to promote coordinated care. Finally, transdisciplinary teams are characterized by role release. More simply stated, team members share roles and responsibilities.

Transdisciplinary teams are known for their family friendliness. In fact, hallmarks of the transdisciplinary structure are equal team status for family members and family-focused consensus-building. Rokusek (1995) notes that the effectiveness of transdisciplinary teams, however, is largely dependent upon discipline comfort and cross-discipline understanding. That said, one of the greatest impediments to success on the transdisciplinary team is difficulty with role release (Landerholm, 1990).

The interdisciplinary team is the final of the three models mentioned in this text and represents middle ground in team functioning. Rokusek (1995) reported several core foundations of interdisciplinary practice including a commitment to one's discipline embedded within a respect for other team members and their contributions, a holistic view of service delivery, a recognition of the interdependent nature of service delivery, and a recognition of cross-disciplinary benefits to consumers.

On the interdisciplinary team, members, including family members, are viewed as equals necessitating equal represenation in decision-making and consensus-building. To accomplish this, interdisciplinary teams work interdependently and collaboratively. Unlike the transdisciplinary team, however, interdisciplinary team members maintain their professional roles. For example, the speech-language pathologist carries primary responsibilities for service delivery specific to communication and language development. It is important to note that even though professional roles are maintained in interdisciplinary functioning, team members must share enough of the knowledge and practices of other disciplines to make appropraite referrals and, in other ways, work together.

Rokusek (1995) identified six abilities needed of members functioning within the interdisciplanary model. First, team members must have an understanding of professional language. This would apply not only to the language of their discipline but other disciplines as well. One of the goals of this text is to expose readers to professional language frequently used by team members. Second, interdisciplinary team members must decrease control of work boundaries while maintaining their professional roles. This allows for interdependency and collaboration. Third, Rokusek noted that interdisciplinary team members must understand and be open to all available service delivery options. Fourth, she suggested that team members must communicate openly and honestly. As will become evident, open and honest communication is a recurring theme of this text. Fifth, interdisciplinary team members must, in the words of Rokusek, "integrate their professional abilities and unique personal qualities into the team, and recognize the specialized culture, values, traditions, knowledge, training, personal emotions, and experiences that the other members bring to the team" (p. 6). Obviously, this type of integration requires a mutual respect that is healthy for any group process. Sixth, interdisciplinary team members must be prepared and willing to work towards consensus building.

Team Characteristics Needed for Optimal Interdisciplinary Functioning

There is a substantial literature on just what makes a team effective. Rather than reviewing this literature in its entirety, what follows is a presentation of seven team characteristics that frequently appear as indicators of effective practice.

Communication

First and foremost, effective teams communicate well. The absence of communication can result in widespread fragmentation of care. Just why do teams need to communicate? Briggs (1993) noted that teams communicate to share information, resolve conflict, discover unique contributions of members, and advocate with administrators and other service providers.

How is communication developed? Communication emerges when team members function within a trusting environment. Only when trust is present do teams begin to take risks as communicators. Such risks might include the forwarding of solutions to problems that are inconsistent with those proposed by other team members. Without the freedom to take risks as communicators, teams do not operate optimally.

Family-Centeredness

One team characteristic generally thought to promote effective practice is family-centeredness. In family-centered practices, family priorities and choices strongly influence service delivery. Dunst, Johanson, Trivette, and Hamby (1991) described a continuum of family-centered services. On one end is professional-centeredness where professionals determine family needs from the professionals' perspectives. Nearer the middle of the continuum is a family-allied perspective where professionals identify family needs and enlist family support to meet those needs. A family-focused approach to teaming encourages families and professionals to work together to determine needs. Once needs are identified, families utilize networks determined by professionals to meet those needs. Finally, in direct contrast to professional-centeredness, a family-centered perspective allows families and professionals to work together to identify and meet needs via family empowerment.

Some might argue that family-centeredness is inconsistent with interdisciplinary practice due to the fact that team members maintain their professional roles. Role identity, then, could be viewed as a deterrent to active family participation in decision-making. The author of this chapter argues, to the contrary, that family-centeredness is a state of mind/action. Accordingly, any team member, including members of interdisciplinary teams, can choose family-centeredness. Making this choice will probably require the weakening of role boundaries mentioned earlier in this chapter.

Familiarity

Landerholm (1990) stated that effective teams develop over time. Therefore, it could be said that one characteristic needed for effective functioning is the familiarity that comes with working together. Familiarity can create a ripe climate for developing communication, trust, and nurturance between and among team members. Of course, familiarity can also lead to poor communication due to assumptions built over time.

Mission

Effective teams have stated missions that reflect the purpose, goals, and philosophy of the team (Briggs, 1993). These missions must emanate from the team as a whole and must be written in ways that team members understand and accept. Pfeiffer (1991) noted that mission statements are most effective if written and revised regularly by the team. This requires a special investment from team members who may find their time limited.

Expertise

Everyone wants team members involved in their care to be experts. Accordingly, we would be remiss to omit expertise as a characteristic of effective teams. Briggs (1993) noted that each team member should bring the following qualities related to expertise to the team: a theoretical and practical knowledge base, strong clinical abilities, and experience with children with disabilities and their families. Obviously, these qualities come from strong preservice preparation and professional experience.

What about families as team members? What expertise can they bring to the team? Families know their member with disabilities better than anyone else. They know what excites and frustrates them. Likewise, they know the roles that this individual plays within their family structure. Parents of older children will not only bring a knowledge of their child to the team, but they may also bring an extensive knowledge of his/her disability.

Support

Effective teams need both internal and external support. Internal support comes from within the team itself. It promotes a trusting environment where communication can occur. It also allows for vulnerability. An internally supportive team allows for members who don't know all the answers and provides assistance when these members need help.

Extenal support is also a characteristic of effective teams. Briggs (1993) noted that teams need resources and autonomy in decision-making. This type of support frequently comes from institutional structures that govern team practice.

Leadership

Finally, strong leadership is critical to effective team practice. For the interdisciplinary team, the team leader will serve in a facilitative role. This might include making sure that all members' issues are addressed equitably, supporting an environment that is trusting and family-centered, and advocating for the family and child with individual team members and other providers. Briggs (1993) noted that an important function of any team leader is the empowerment of other team members to lead.

Families as Team Members

A discussion of families as team members should probably begin by noting that families don't ask for disability. Accordingly, their service on interdisciplinary or other teams is something they haven't prepared for—something they never expected to do. That said, family members can grow into effective and empowered team players. This growth, however, is dependent upon caring professionals and families' and the professionals' willingness to learn.

Lubetsky, Mueller, Madden, Walker, and Len (1995) provided an interesting discussion of families as team members. These authors noted that a first step to the effective service of family members on teams is engagement in the team process. What is engagement? It would appear that for Lubetsky et al., engagement refers to active involvement. They stated that engagement "helps to align [families] with professionals from many disciplines, empowers them, and maintains their responsibility in decision-making" (Lubetsky et al., 1995; p. 254).

One could argue that families' engagement with team activities should be preceded by, or at least coexist with, an educational effort specific to team processes and team members' roles. For example, it would seem that preliminary efforts to convey the team's mission and the expertise of members would be appropriate. It would also seem fruitful to convey typical roles that families may be asked to play. This sharing could be organized by the team leader. Of course, family members should be allowed to contribute to, and alter the team's mission from their perspective. Likewise, families should be encouraged to share openly their levels of team participation and ultimate expectations. Hopefully, this open sharing will result in an integrated and mutually agreed upon team plan. Leviton, Mueller, and Kauffman (1992) suggested that family-professional dialog assists with the team plan by determining the family-professional relationship, setting team goals, generating strategies to meet goals, and constructing teams for service delivery.

Once family engagement has occurred, family members are often asked to contribute to the team process as informants. As was mentioned earlier in this chapter, families know more about their child with a disability than anyone else does. This information is critical to effective team practice. For example, knowledge of prior medical procedures can have significant implications regarding assessment and treatment decisions. Likewise, knowing that time with a computer game is rewarding to a child might be very useful to professionals needing reinforcers to complete standardized assessment or encourage particpation in treatment activities.

Aside from serving as informants, family members will most probably be asked to evaluate the representativeness of their child's responses during assessment or treatment procedures. Without family feedback, other team members only have their observations to guide decision making. Unfortunately, these observations may not reflect reality. Family members can play a vital role in conveying how closely the behaviors observed during clinical activities represent reality as it is perceived by those close to the child. This kind of information can be very useful when determining developmental status or progress.

Finally, Lubetsky et al. (1995) noted that family members often serve as extensions of the assessment or treatment team. For example, parents or siblings may be asked to interact with the child during an assessment. Likewise, parents, grandparents, siblings, and others may be trained in therapeutic and medical techniques to assist with the generalization of skills beyond clinical training contexts and to promote good health.

In considering all the potential roles of family members, teams must remember the concept of family-centeredness. Simply stated, teams should be focused primarily upon encouraging an environment where family members feel comfortable and confident contributing in every way.

Tips for Beginning the Team Process

The tips shared below come from Robert Fulghum's (1989) book *All I Really Need to Know I Learned in Kindergarten.* This timeless little book holds wisdom for all who aspire to function optimally as team members. Each tip is provided with a brief discussion of its application to team functioning.

Share Everything

When it comes to information, interdisciplinary teams must be interdependent. Team interdependence requires an openness with respect to knowledge, expectations, goals, and dreams. It is largely dependent upon a willingness to spend the time together necessary for familiarity and learning.

As those of us who are parents know, sharing doesn't come easy. Professionals have largely been trained to "own" their knowledge. Therefore, sharing will require some effort. Likewise, families may have had painful experiences specific to their child's care. Recounting these experiences can also be difficult. A commitment to open and honest communication should be the answer to effective sharing.

Play Fair

Most teams inevitably experience some negative dynamics during team processes. Fatigue, dominance by one member, and overstatements of findings can lead to fractionation and bad feelings. An initial commitment to respect each team member's contributions will promote positive team interactions. Furthermore, an understanding that members have a common goal, e.g., the welfare of the child and family, should encourage tolerance during difficult times.

Remember... The First Word You Learned - The Biggest Word of All - LOOK

Too often, team members fall into the trap of discipline absorption. We get so consumed with our concerns that we fail to see the whole child and family. By taking time to look and communicate, teams will be more holistic and more effective.

Warm Cookies and Cold Milk Are Good for You

Few teams take time to bask in their success. In contrast, almost all teams agonize over their failures. A few minutes to reflect on successes can be both supportive to team members and serve a useful function of follow-up with families.

In sum, you have to work at being an effective team. A final tip from Fulghum (1994) tells it all. If teams "watch out for traffic, hold hands, and stick together" (p. 35), they will serve well. It is the authors' hope that this brief introduction to teaming has provided the basic tools to do just that.

REFERENCES

Ackerly, A. (1947). The clinic team. *American Journal of Orthopsychiatry, 17*, 191-195.

Allen, K.E., Holm, V.A., & Schiefelbusch, R.L. (Eds). (1978). *Early intervention: A team approach.* Baltimore: University Park Press.

Beck, H.L., (1962). The advantages of a multi-purpose clinic for the mentally retarded. *American Journal of Mental Deficiency, 66*, 789-794.

Briggs, M.H. (1993). Team talk: Communication skills for early intervention teams. *Journal of Childhood Communication Disorders, 15* (1), 33-40.

Dunst, C.J., Johanson, C., Trivette, C.M., & Hamby, D. (1991). Family-oriented early intervnetion poliecies and practices. Family-centered or not? *Exceptional Children, 58*, 115-126.

Fulghum, R. (1994). *All I really need to know I learned in kindergarten.* New York: Villard.

Golin, A.K., and Ducanis, A.J. (1981). *The interdisciplinary team.* Rockville, MD: Aspen.

Hart, V. (1977). The use of many disciplines with the severely and profoundly handicapped. in E. Sontag, J. Smith, & N. Certo (Eds.), *Educational programming for the severely and profoundly handicapped.* Reston, VA: Division on Mental Retardation, Council on Exceptional Children.

Landerholm, E. (1990). The transdisciplinary team approach in infant programs. *Teaching Exceptional Children*, 66-70.

Leviton, A., Mueller, M., & Kauffman, C. (1992). The family-centered-consultation model: Practical applications for professionals. *Infants and Young Children, 4* (3), 1-8.

Lubetsky, M.J., Mueller, L., Madden, K., Walker, R., & Len, D. (1995). Family-centered/interdisciplinary team approach to working with families of children who have mental retardation. *Mental Retardation, 33* (4), 251-256.

Lyon, S., & Lyon, G. (1980). Team functioning and staff development: A role release approach to providing educational services for severely handicapped students. *Journal of the Association for the Severely Handicapped, 5*, 250-263.

Pfeiffer, J.W. (Ed.) (1991). *The encyclopedia of team-development activities.* San Diego, CA: Pfeiffer.

Rokusek, C. (1995). An introduction to the concept of interdisciplinary practice. In B. Thyer and N. Kropf (Eds.). *Developmental disabilities: A handbook for interdisciplinary practice* (p. 1 - 12). Cambridge, MA: Brookline.

Chapter 2

THE PARENT-PROFESSIONAL RELATIONSHIP

JANE B. SCHULZ AND MARTIN A. FISCHER

Billy was 18 months old before we had a diagnosis of Down syndrome. He was our third child, and we recognized the delayed development. Our physician insisted that he would "be all right" and that we were over-anxious parents. Our frustration increased as we became more and more concerned about Billy's slow development. We didn't know what to do or how to explain his behavior to family, to friends, and to ourselves. After moving to a larger city, we found a good pediatrician who gave us the proper diagnosis.

In contrast, Ross (1993) describes the trauma of early discovery when her physician came into the hospital room after her delivery and announced, "Mrs. Ross, your baby has Down's [Down] syndrome." She relates that

> Years later, talking with other parents of babies who were mentally retarded, I would discuss whether it is easier to learn of the baby's disability all at once or little by little. Whether the hard, quick blow bleeds less and heals faster than the slow, gnawing fear that something is wrong but no one will come out and say exactly what. After thirty years, I still don't know the answer, except that there is no easy way. (p. 19)

Regardless of the timing or the manner of delivery of the news, families of children with disabilities are placed in a unique position. Not only are they faced with the pressures and responsibilities that all children present, but they have the added challenge of integrating a child with disabilities into the life and the social structure of the family. In attempting to deal with a difficult situation, parents have turned to professionals in the fields of medicine, education, and related areas for help. The direction of this help has changed dramatically over the past twenty-five years.

Parents of children with disabilities were recipients of services long before they became participants in designing and implementing such services. As

12

recipients, they were frequently served within the clinical model, a model that traditionally has viewed children with disabilities, and therefore their parents, as patients. This model, which is used by social workers, therapists, psychologists, and physicians, operates under the assumption that treatment will be determined solely by professionals.

As parents and other family members became advocates for their children with disabilities, they also revealed dissatisfaction with their lack of involvement in the evaluation and treatment process. They felt that meaningful communication between parents and professionals was difficult, if not impossible, and that parents were granted little respect by the professionals who were dictating their children's programs. One mother stated the position of many parents in the following passage:

> . . . I am clearly one of the lost generation of parents of handicapped children. We are parents who are either intimidated by professionals or angry with them, or both; parents who are unreasonably awed by them; parents who intuitively know that we know our children better than the experts of any discipline and yet we persistently assume that the professionals know best; parents who carry so much attitudinal and emotional baggage around with us that we are unable to engage in any real dialogue with professionals–teachers, principals, physicians, or psychologists-about our children. (Gorham, 1975, p. 521)

It became increasingly clear that the parent-professional relationship was not only an inadequate one, it was also an adversarial one. Attitudes contributing to this poor relationship include negative stereotyping of parents, blaming parents for the child's problems, furnishing inadequate information, and exhibiting nonaccepting attitudes toward parents (Schulz, 1987). Fox (1979) explained the resultant poor relationship:

> Whenever parents of handicapped children meet or talk together, a frequent topic of conversation is the perceived lack of empathy and understanding by "professionals" of the parents' concerns, pressures and goals for their children. Some parents react to this so strongly that individual meetings with professionals and group staffings become major traumatic events to be dreaded and avoided. (p. 36)

A constant theme in the literature during the 1970s is the inclination of professionals not to listen to parents nor to accept their input concerning their child with a disability. Seligman (1970) describes this proclivity: "There is a tendency for professionals to discount whatever parents say about their child, as professionals believe that their perceptions are the only valid ones and that parents' observations are colored by subjectivity, denial, or distortions of reality" (p. 139).

Professionals who work with children who have disabilities have been almost as verbal as parents in expressing their difficulties with the relationship. Problem areas include parents' dependency, unrealistic expectations, antagonism toward professional people, and role conflict.

One professional, in seeing the parent as an adversary, explained that

> Sometimes, parents adopt an adversarial role when they seek services that may be unreasonable, dismiss alternatives that may be appropriate though less costly, and stridently advocate for their children. Professionals who have been "burned" by experiences of this kind begin to approach parents warily, expecting the worst. Unfortunately, this attitude can be very destructive to a new relationship. (Sonnenschein, 1981, p. 64)

I became aware of both perspectives when, already the parent of a child with Down syndrome, I became a special education teacher. During a conference with the mother of a child in my class, we were discussing the child's progress and needs. She suddenly railed out, "You teachers don't know anything about these children!" Although I wanted to say to her, "I understand how you feel," I also resented her implications, knowing that I had spent a great deal of time with her child and cared deeply about his education.

Regardless of the circumstances, roles of parents and professionals have been separated by philosophies, education, experience, and environment. Traditionally, the different perspectives have been viewed as "sides"–a tragic status in determining what is best for the person with the disability.

With the passage and implementation of Public Law 94-142 (changed to Individuals with Disabilities Act or IDEA), it became clear that the role of the parent was to be an active, participating one. The effects of parent advocacy through organized groups and individual pressures are clearly expressed in each section of this law. Evaluation of the child and development of the Individual Education Program require full participation by the parent. While all parents are not involved in the process, whether by choice or circumstances, the opportunity and responsibility are provided and fostered.

Turnbull and Turnbull (1997) define the role of parents as collaborators as distinguished from that as decision makers or as recipients of professionals' judgments. As collaborators, the assumption is made that families will be "equal and full partners with educators and school systems and that this collaboration will affect the student and school system operations as well" (p. 11). They stress the individuality of parents in the assumption of their roles and identify dimensions of the change that has occurred. The first dimension of change moves from viewing parents as part of the child's problem to viewing them as collaborators in addressing the challenges of exceptionality.

Second, they shift from insisting on passive roles for parents to expecting active and collaborating roles for families. Further, they strive to recognize the preferences and needs of all members of a family, rather than viewing families as a mother-child dyad. Finally, they attempt to respond to families individually as a whole and for each member of the family instead of responding to family needs in a general way (p. 12).

As professionals in the field of special education and as the parent of an individual with a disability, we (the editors) wondered if parents had become collaborators and team members and if they were satisfied with the current parent-professional relationship. As a means of providing authors of the discipline-specific chapters with parent concerns and questions, a national/international survey was conducted, using *The Bridging the Family-Professional Gap Family Member Survey.*

THE SURVEY

The Bridging the Family-Professional Gap Family Member Survey was created by a graduate student at Western Carolina University with input from the editors and under their supervision. It was designed to allow parents or other family members to describe themselves and their family member with a disability, to convey their perceptions of the professional services received by their family member, and to voice comments and questions directly to professionals working in various disciplines.

Section A of the survey sought family demographic information in a checklist and short answer format. Using a similar format, Section B requested a description of the individual with a disability, the nature and severity of the disability, and the family environment. In this section, the caregiver was asked to describe the family's entry into the human services system and to describe initial contacts with professionals as well as events related to receiving a diagnosis of disability for their family member. Caregivers were also asked to indicate the nature of the services provided to date, including whether their family has been served by teams or by individual practitioners. Section B concluded with questions specific to the length of time services had been provided, the nature of current services, the relative ease of acquiring services, and the resources which have been of the greatest help to the family.

Section C presented open-ended questions to allow respondents the opportunity to discuss service-related issues and to raise questions or make comments for professionals.

Finally, Section D presented a series of Likert-scale items that provide information about whether respondents perceive professionals to be operating according to the principles of family-centeredness. A copy of the survey is provided in the Appendix and can be obtained from the editors.

Survey Distribution

In the spring of 1997, 250 hard copies of *The Bridging the Family-Professional Gap* survey and self-addressed envelopes were distributed to parent advocacy organizations in California, Colorado, Kansas, Massachusetts, North Carolina, Oregon, and Texas. These seven states were selected to represent the major geographic regions of the United States. Advocacy groups were chosen at random from internet web sites. A deliberate effort was made to include both rural and urban groups. Prior to mailing surveys, telephone calls were made to each advocacy group explaining the book's premise and requesting assistance with the distribution and return of surveys. Participating advocacy groups were also encouraged to photocopy and circulate additional copies of the survey as widely as possible.

By early summer of 1997, the survey was also placed on the World Wide Web. The survey was linked electronically to over 100 related web sites, including home pages of national organizations serving parents and families with children with disabilities and personal home pages of parents of children with disabilities. In addition, all chapter authors were asked to distribute the survey's web address.

All surveys (both hard and electronic copies) included an informed consent section which, if completed by the respondent, would allow survey contents to be used in this book.

Survey Returns and Descriptions of Respondents

By late fall of 1997, 34 hard copy surveys and 464 electronic surveys had been returned. Surveys were returned from 49 of the United States and 13 other countries. The majority of respondents were Caucasian (92%) mothers (86%) who described themselves as primary caregivers (83%) of their child with a disability. Most respondents reported that they had received either graduate level education (17%), college education (66%), or high school education (7%). Respondents' occupations were extremely varied and included homemaking, teaching, sales, corporate training, accounting, office management, and nursing. Most respondents (81%) reported that a two-parent family best described their structure.

Over half of the respondents (59%) reported that their family member with a disability was male with ages of the family member ranging from one month to 53 years old. Most family members lived at home (94% and most were the youngest child in the family (41%). The greatest number of the family members with a disability were between the ages of birth to three years, many from 10 to 20 and a few from 20 to 41. Respondents reported a wide array of conditions when asked to describe the nature of their child's disability. The most frequent responses included autism, mental retardation, speech and language delay, learning disability, orthopedic impairment, emotional and behavior impairment, seizure disorder, and visual impairment. Other responses included attention deficit disorder, traumatic brain injury, and brain disorder. Most respondents described their child as having moderate or severe disabilities, with some indicating mild disabilities. A summary of information specific to family members with disabilities is provided in

Table 2-1

	General Information	
Number of Surveys Returned	464	
Number of States	49	
Number of Countries	13	
	Respondent Information	
Relation to Child with Disability		
Mother	400	(86%)
Father	45	(10%)
Other	19	(4%)
Ethnicity		
African American	5	(1%)
Asian American	5	(1%)
Caucasian	428	(92%)
Hispanic American	5	(1%)
Other	21	(5%)
Education		
Elementary School	18	(4%)
Some High School	60	(13%)
Some College	306	(66%)
Graduate Degree	78	(17%)
	Person with Disability	
Gender		
Male	272	(62%)
Female	166	(38%)

Age

Less than 1 year	21	(4%)
1-3 years	107	(23%)
4-5 years	90	(19%)
6-12 years	171	(36%)
13-21 years	62	(13%)
Older than 21 years	21	(4%)

Location in Family

Only child	116	(25%)
Youngest child	188	(41%)
Middle child (or one of middle)	57	(13%)
Oldest child	103	(22%)

Lives at home

Yes	434	(97%)
No	14	(3%)

Primary Disability

Autism	97	(21%)
Orthopedic Impairment	25	(5%)
Emotional/Behavioral Impairment	1	(<1%)
Speech/Language Impairment	37	(8%)
Hearing Impairment	23	(5%)
Visual Impairment	10	(2%)
Learning Disability	29	(6%)
Mental Retardation	46	(10%)
Other	197	(42%)

Description of Responses

In describing the family's entry into the human services system and services provided, the caregivers reported that most children were diagnosed from birth to two years (72%), some from three years to nine years (27%), and a few from 10 years to 14 years (2%). The initial diagnoses were made primarily by physicians (33%) and psychologists (7%). Professionals involved in planning or delivery of services predominately included audiologist, counselor, dentist, neurologist, nurse, nutritionist, occupational therapist, physical therapist, physician, psychologist, social worker, special educator, and speech-language pathologist. Professionals listed most frequently as primary providers of services were occupational therapist, physical therapist, physician, special educator, and speech-language pathologist. Family members are served almost equally by individual professionals and by a team of professionals and the majority are currently enrolled in educational programs. The number of years the family member has received special services ranges from none to 20 years. The family members are served by individual professionals (56%) and by teams of professionals (36%). Nearly all the family

members are currently enrolled in educational programs (76%). A summary
of information related to family members with disabilities is presented in

Table 2-2

Age of Diagnosis		
Less than 1 year	245	(53%)
1-3 years	135	(29%)
4-5 years	52	(11%)
6-12 years	23	(5%)
13-21 years	7	(2%)
Older than 21 years	2	(<1%)
Initial Diagnosis Made By		
Audiologist	39	(8%)
Nurse	1	(<1%)
Physician	152	(33%)
Speech-Language Pathologist	29	(6%)
Psychologist	33	(7%)
ENT	8	(2%)
Occupational Therapist	3	(<1%)
Social Worker	3	(<1%)
Self	27	(6%)
Neurologist	74	(16%)
Physical Therapist	2	(<1%)
Special Educator	8	(2%)
Other	85	(18%)
Professional Involved in Planning and Delivery		
Audiologist	196	(42%)
Nurse	156	(34%)
Physician	374	(81%)
Speech-Language Pathologist	334	(72%)
Psychologist	189	(41%)
ENT	281	(61%)
Occupational Therapist	310	(67%)
Social Worker	182	(39%)
Neurologist	244	(53%)
Physical Therapist	261	(56%)
Special Educator	316	(68%)
Other	112	(24%)
Served by		
Individual Professional	261	(59%)
Team of Professionals	165	(37%)
Both	18	(4%)
Years Served		
Less than 1 year	62	(14%)
1-3 years	164	(38%)
4-5 years	60	(14%)
6-12 years	102	(24%)
13-21 years	40	(9%)
More than 21 years	2	(<1%)

Description of Services

The majority of families found that services were available in their communities and that it was not necessary to relocate the family. As indicated in Table 2-3, the types of communities represented ranged from rural to suburban, with more families living in suburban areas.

Table 2-3

Type of Community		
Rural	91	(20%)
Suburban	209	(45%)
Small City	123	(27%)
Large City	41	(9%)

The respondents were most concerned about what to tell people and found that the immediate and extended family was their greatest resource. In response to questions about interactions with professionals, the *majority* of respondents *agreed* with statements in Figure 2-1; *agreed somewhat* with statements in Figure 2-2; and *disagreed* with statements in Figure 2-3.

Figure 2-1

The majority of respondents <u>agreed</u> with the following statements:

- Professionals have a good understanding of the family member's disability.
- They understand the family member's disability.
- The program the family member is in has helped the family understand the problem better.
- Professionals address their questions and concerns in a straightforward manner.
- Technical terms used by the professionals are explained to them.
- The information about the family member's disability was presented in understandable terms.
- Adequate information was given about the family member's disability.
- Professionals asked for their opinions and suggestions concerning the family member's disability.
- Professionals fully informed them about the family member's disability, current level of functioning, and outlook for the future.
- The responsibilities of each team member were fully explained.
- Professionals treated the family with compassion.

- Professionals were honest and sincere.
- Professionals viewed the family in a positive light.
- Professionals valued the family's knowledge, opinions, and observations.
- Professionals' advice was worth following.
- Family members had regular contact with professionals.
- The program the family member is in seems to be helping.
- Family members had regular contact with professionals.

Figure 2-2

The majority of respondents <u>agreed somewhat</u> with the following statements:

- Professionals focused on understanding the needs and priorities of the family.
- The needs and priorities of the family set the direction for treatment.
- Professionals provided support by helping the family make its own decisions about needed services and intervention goals.

Figure 2-3

The majority of respondents <u>disagreed</u> with the following statements:

- It was easy to get help for the family member.
- Professionals helped them learn new skills to get resources to meet their needs.
- The team helped them learn new skills to get resources to meet their needs.
- All the professionals on the team were equally helpful.

For the purpose of this survey, responses to the open-ended questions provided the most interesting information and directions for change in the parent-professional relationship and team functioning.

Respondents' Questions and Comments

Respondents were asked to give us comments to pass on to professionals: questions for team members, advice to professionals, services they would seek if they were to start over, and the aspect of their family member's disability that has been most difficult to deal with. The responses in all four categories mainly dealt with encouraging professionals to listen to the families, urging the improvement of team collaboration, asking for suggestions on ways families could help their members with disabilities, asking for respect and honesty from professionals, seeking more information about services, and looking for support groups and systems. Some of the questions posed and comments made are included in Figure 2-4.

Figure 2-4
QUESTIONS AND COMMENTS

Listen To Me

- Listen to family members and hear them. Professionals are with our children for a little while; we are there 24 hours a day, 7 days a week.
- Why do you fight me so hard when I tell you there's a problem? Why can't you trust my instincts and the knowledge I have about my children?
- Remember that parents know their children better than anyone and most of the time the choices they make are right for them.
- Respect the fact that parents know their children best, including their needs, appropriate services, and levels of care. Invite the professionals to care for their special needs child one week and see if their opinions change.
- Look at each client as an individual and listen to caregivers.
- Ask parents more for input.
- Believe that the parent knows what she speaks about. Try some of the parent's ideas—they just might work.
- Make a conscious effort to hear and not be so quick to form an opinion.

Team Collaboration

- Talk to each other.
- We have worked with many caring and competent professionals. The main problems are due to lack of service coordination, and lack of collaboration among agencies and services. Families become exhausted by the "run-around" delays, red-tape, insurance discrimination, etc.
- Family members are a valuable member of the team, but we must also allow individuals who have disabilities and are able to speak out and teach. I think people should be more involved or the services we have may cease to exist.
- Please learn how to better work with family members; they are part of the team.

- Why do so many mental health professionals not actively advocate for better and adequate mental health systems of care? Family advocates need help and support.
- Training should be given to team members.
- We have been very fortunate with the team of professionals that work with our son at his school. They have been great trying different techniques and strategies to help him learn as much as possible.

Suggest Ways I Can Help

- Outline a course of action for my son. Teach me to teach him at home.
- Many families need guidance promptly after diagnosis is given. Outline successive steps with them. It's hard enough dealing with the grief without worrying what to do next.
- Try different approaches. What works for one individual doesn't always have the same effect on others. Have a lot of follow up. Concentrate on issues that will be useful to the client.

Respect and Honesty

- Respect families—all families.
- It's OK to be human. It's OK to cry with me.
- Be open and up front at all times; good and bad parents have a right to know everything.
- Please stop putting us on hold and saying "maybe." Please give us the truth and facts.
- Do not speak in front of our children with disabilities as if they don't understand what you're saying.
- The only bad experience we have had has been with physicians making judgments or inappropriate comments. I think all medical students should be required to pass a class on bedside manners.
- If my child shows regressions, don't imply that something I did or am doing has caused it. Just because I am more emotional, worried, or depressed than usual doesn't mean this is the case. Regressed behaviors in children can bring on regressed behaviors in parents. Remember that parenting children with disabilities is very challenging.
- Some professionals seem to lose a sense of compassion for the individual and family. The sensitivity to the situation is lost and a "what did you expect" attitude begins. This has been difficult for me.
- Respect the parent and the knowledge they have about their child. When the child is placed out of the home, remember the parent is still the guardian or double check that the parent is getting the information.

• Try to involve the family in all situations and be understanding of our situations at home. Give us encouragement for trying to comply with all the treatments that are so overwhelming. Honestly care. We are fed up with "you're just the parent" syndrome.

Seeking Information

• Why aren't families given special education law information? I could tell horror stories about children not getting services!
• Write down all information you give to parents so that when they come home, they can read over the information later. Relate testing and instructions so it is in a language or words that parents can relate to.
• We were not given financial information in the beginning: Medicaid, crippled children's, shriner's, etc. I did my own research for resources which was very difficult. Every family should be given state information on special education laws, etc., upon diagnosis.
• I'm lucky that I had the education and gumption to fight. Many parents, especially low income or low education, would not even know where to start. No one should have to fight and blindly forge around looking for services and they should be offered information without having to know the right questions to ask.

Looking for Support

• The parent support group has been our greatest source of information and a place to share our common grief. We didn't have a support group initially, but we found others and formed one.
• If I were starting over I would look sooner for the parent support groups and encourage others to do the same. Other parents understand better what you're going through, and give great advice on what works and what doesn't.
• Parent support groups and social gatherings have been very therapeutic for us.
• Communication with other families is the best way to educate us all.
• If professionals could link up families with similarly disabled children, it would be helpful.
• If professionals aren't able to help the situation, they should refer the child to someone who can. If available, refer them to a support group where they can get ideas from others. Support is vital!
• Support groups are very helpful if disabilities are as severe as your child's. Sponsor families to attend national, regional, and local confer-

ences. This was invaluable to us. They are usually too expensive for the family to afford. Our child lives for the week of camp each year that is for her particular disability. The medical team helps with this.

- Why does it have to be so hard? Everything I've done in connection with my child's disability has been difficult, from finding a diagnostician, to all the testing, to the search for information in countless books and articles, to the working through the grief process, and much more.
- Just because a parent is a professional and has a decent income, why is it so difficult to get services? Because my son is not the "squeaky wheel" why do I have to fight so hard for services?
- What are universities involved in training teachers doing to insure that regular education teachers will recognize children who learn differently so they can be referred for help as soon as possible?
- Why can't programs be more preventive rather than waiting until crisis occurs?

If Respondents Were to Start Over, They Would Seek the Following Services:

- A pediatrician who understands children with special needs.
- More speech/language help.
- Kindergarten screening for LD.
- Speech-language pathologist, OT, psychologist, audiologist, private tutors or private school.
- I would educate myself first. Second, I would seek more parent groups.
- I would have sought services earlier. And not be afraid of using medications.
- I would learn more about my son's disability and be more assertive about services needed.
- Focus on positive behaviors rather than negative actions/behaviors of my child.
- More integration with non-disabled people.
- Begin my own research rather than rely on the system.
- Education.
- Respite services.
- Accurate drug information.
- I wish I'd known when he was in preschool. I'd have had different expectations and gotten psycho-motor skills assistance.
- Same services; I just know now where to go and how to expedite things.
- Counseling specific to my son's needs.
- I've gotten what I need but it's been a battle.

The respondents specified the conditions in Figure 2-5 as the aspect of their family member's disability that has been most difficult to deal with. Perhaps the most relevant feature of the survey results in advice that care-givers offer to professionals who work with chldren with disabilities and their families. Samples of this advice are provided in Figure 2-6.

Figure 2-5
MOST DIFFICULT CONDITIONS TO DEAL WITH

- The emotional part.
- Stress of repeated fractures/multiple surgeries.
- Dual diagnosis—coordinating services (a nightmare).
- Uncertain potential failure.
- Inability to fully communicate.
- Seeing the difference between the eldest son and the three younger.
- The learning disability.
- Mood swings, frustration, ANGER.
- Difficult to deal with fact that she may not go any further cognitively.
- Future uncertainties. Slowness of the process getting him diagnosed and placed. Heartache of an abnormal child—grief.
- I feel bad about the fact that my daughter with Down syndrome will not get to do the same things my older daughter will get to do.
- My autistic son's behaviors and rigidness—trying to explain this to others.
- The constant regression of skills.
- How she perceives herself, how her self-esteem is affected. Coping strategies for her.
- I have many people to help my child when he is in school and no one to help me treat him normally at home.
- Her physical handicaps have been the most difficult for us. We are a very active family and all participate in a wide variety of sports. We can never do this as a family as someone has to stay home with our child with a disability.
- Mood swings—hard for her and for us.
- Toilet training—lack of it.
- Other people's judgments of me as a mother based on his behavior.
- The loss of potential in such an intelligent, talented human being due to her no-fault brain disorder.
- School personnel are very hard to work with. Treatments are very time-consuming. Feel guilty to spend time doing anything else. Our family is

very stressed, depressed, sad, lonely, feel helpless, etc. Family and church, neighbors, friends don't understand or care. IEP's are very difficult and stressful.
- Bad behaviors.
- Being a single parent and not knowing how to deal with behavior.

Figure 2-6
ADVICE TO PROFESSIONALS

- Train all teachers about LD. Test to identify early. Include parents and the student in discussions regarding appropriate services, modifications, etc.
- Please try to stay informed, so that you can give parents good information.
- Advise parents of all options available for treatment of their child's disability.
- Recommend services available in the community.
- Be compassionate.
- Learn more about disabilities, and keep up with the literature. Also, work closely with the parents (who know their child so well) and encourage them not to give up on their unending efforts to do what's best for the child.
- Be aware of all resources and make them available.
- Put yourself in the parent's place 24 hours a day. Be patient. Don't just do what you have to do. Go the extra mile. Help put parents and clients in touch with the services.
- We have had a mixture of good, bad, and mediocre professionals working with our children. The good are worth their weight in gold. The bad have caused us more pain than we deserve. The mediocre have been entirely too forgettable. I would like for professionals to top and think about the one person they love most in the world and how they would like to hear information about that person before they ever open their mouths to speak to a parent who has a child with special needs.

Certainly there have been positive changes in the parent-professional relationship. One parent made the following comment:

> We have been very fortunate with the team of professionals that work with our son at this school. They have been great trying different techniques and strategies to help him learn as much as possible.

Another parent expresses appreciation in the following comment:

> I would like to say that I owe deep gratitude to the early professionals who were involved in my son's specific needs. Many of them spoke up for my son when I did not have enough knowledge and understanding to do it alone. They gave me the little nudge and encouragement that I needed to make some important decisions about my son's future.

ANALYSIS OF THE SURVEY

In examining the responses to *The Bridging the Family-Professional Gap* survey, we find that the participants do not represent an average group of parents. The demographic information shows parents who are mainly female, Caucasian, from two-parent homes, with occupations in moderate to high level positions. The family members with disabilities are young, with a few to age 20 and none over 41 and have severe to moderate disabilities. It is also important to acknowledge that the respondents have access to and use computers and have average to high educational levels.

Although this group does not appear to be representative of families who have children with disabilities, it is representative of parents who are advocates for their family members. As one parent expressed it, "I'm lucky that I had the education and gumption to fight. Many parents, especially low income or low education, would not even know where to start." Thus the concerns and questions posed by this group can be extrapolated to other families and to their children who have disabilities. In summary, the respondents are addressing the following issues: They are asking professionals to listen to parents, urging use of the team approach, asking professionals to give them strategies and suggestions, and requesting professionals to be patient with them and their child. They also are asking that professionals show respect for the family and to be honest with them, stressing the importance of support groups, and requesting that professionals give them accurate and full information.

In looking at parent observations in the 1970s and 1980s, we find many of the same concerns. During that period, Gliedman and Roth (1980) examined the roles of parents and professionals in an attempt to understand the conflicts in their relationships. They point out the vast asymmetry in need between the parent and the professional and emphasize that in most cases the parent needs the professional far more than the professional needs any one parent. They also acknowledge that the parent is focused on one child, while the professional has many children as clients; further, the professional does not have the emotional commitment to the child that the parent has. This point is made clear in subsequent chapters and is an understandable barrier. While the work of parent groups and the influence of IDEA in requiring parent participation in the educational process has brought about some reform, it is clear that the gap continues to exist. Collaboration is also difficult between and among professionals who are involved in the diagnosis and treatment of children with disabilities. Sedlak (1997) states that "the alliance between schools and the mental health services provided by social workers, counselors, and experts in guidance and child welfare has always been uneasy" (p. 349). However, the effective collaboration of educational and health care professionals on behalf of children with special needs was never more clearly mandated than in the passage of IDEA.

In discussing the hospital as an important site for family-centered early intervention, Long, Artis, and Dobbins (1993) admit that although the diverse professionals from the health care and early intervention fields may have the common goal of family-centered care, collaboration between programs presents challenges. They offer guidelines for effective collaboration. Effective communication is vital to a collaborative partnership. In a hospital setting, communication can take place during team meetings, telephone contacts, and letters, while information can be shared through chart documentation and developmental play plans. Families of children who are hospitalized for longer periods of time are increasingly interested in information to enhance their child's development. The IFSP (Individualized Family Service Plan) process is an excellent means for providing this information. Parents find support through meeting other parents of children with similar needs. Parent-to-parent support groups in hospitals are one way of assisting family-centered care. A single hospital contact improves cooperation between community-based early intervention services and hospital staff. Training in family-centered care practices must be ongoing in a hospital setting due to the nature of the institution and its staffing patterns (p.117).

P.L. 99-457, Education of the Handicapped Amendments, redefined the concept of family involvement as well as collaboration among professionals in the educational process by identifying families, not just children, as the recipients of services. In search for responses to this legislative challenge, early interventionists have turned to the child health domain and have embraced the family-centered philosophy. The basic tenets of family-centered philosophy require a collaborative relationship wherein professionals do things with, not to, families (Baird & Peterson, 1997).

The most obvious statement of a family focus in P.L. 99-457 is the requirement for an Individualized Family Service Plan (IFSP) for programs serving infants and toddlers. Assumptions arising out of models dealing with the family-centered approach in early childhood education would serve to bridge the gap observed at all levels. Children and families are inextricably intertwined. Intentional or not, intervention with children almost invariably influences families; likewise, intervention with and support of families almost invariably influence children. Involving and supporting families is likely to be a more powerful intervention than one that focuses exclusively on the child. Family members should be able to choose their level of involvement in program planning, decision-making, and service delivery. Professionals should attend to family priorities for goals and services, even when those priorities differ substantially from professional priorities (Bailey, Buysse, Edmondson, & Smith, 1992, p. 298).

Although the most outstanding efforts promoting full collaboration appear to be evident in early childhood programs, we can learn a great deal from researching programs dealing with diverse populations of children with special needs. An example is Project STAR, an early intervention program developed in response to concerns of families who have children with AIDS in their homes (Woodruff, 1994). The needs of these parents were similar to those stated in *The Bridging the Family-Professional Gap Family Member Survey*. The family is recognized as the primary and most significant force in the child's life and the goal for professionals is to support, not supplant, the role of the family. The role of the staff in this project is stated as follows:

> Staff accept families as they are, build on their strengths, respond to their priorities for services even when they differ from staff objectives, respect their different methods for coping, and build a strong parent-to-parent peer support component that offers parents the opportunity to build friendships and get the kind of support that only parents can provide for one another. (p. 45)

As parents and professionals, we have much to learn from each other.

It is the hope of the authors of this book that putting families in closer touch with the professionals involved with their children will facilitate communication with and respect for each other. Serving children who have disabilities and their families is more than a legal issue: it is a human issue. Collaboration is the answer.

REFERENCES

Bailey, D. B., Buysse, V., Edmondson, R., & Smith, T. (1992). Creating family-centered services in early intervention: Perceptions of professionals in four states. *Exceptional Children, 54* (4), 298-308.

Baird, S., & Peterson, J. (1997). Seeking a comfortable fit between family-centered philosophy and infant-parent interaction in early intervention: Time for a paradigm shift? *Topics in Early Childhood Special Education, 17* (2), 139-164.

Fox, D. C. (1979). Parents teach professionals. *Education Unlimited, 1* (5), 36-37.

Gliedman, J., & Roth, W. (1980). *The unexpected minority*. New York: Harcourt Brace Jovanovich.

Gorham, K. A. (1975). A lost generation of parents. *Exceptional Children, 41* (8), 521-525.

Long, C. E., Artis, N. E., & Dobbins, N. J. (1993). The hospital: An important site for family-centered early intervention. *Topics in Early Childhood Special Education 13* (1), 106-119.

Ross, B. M. (1993). *Our special child.* Nashville, TN: Thomas Nelson.

Schulz, J. B. (1987). *Parents and professionals in special education.* New York: Allyn and Bacon.

Sedlak, M. W. (1997). The uneasy alliance of mental health services and the schools: An historical perspective. *American Orthopsychiatric Association, Inc, 67* (3), 349-362).

Seligman, M. (1979). *Strategies for helping parents of handicapped children.* New York: Free Press.

Sonnenschein, P. (1981). Parents and professionals: An uneasy relationship. *Teaching Exceptional Children, 14* (2), 62-65.

Turnbull, A. P., & Turnbull, H. R. (1997). *Families, professionals, and exceptionality* (3rd ed.). Upper Saddle River, N: Merrill.

Woodruff, G. (1994). Serving the needs of children with AIDS and their families. *Teaching Exceptional Children, 26* (4), 45-47.

Chapter 3

MEDICINE

BLAIR M. EIG

As a pediatrician and the father of a son who has a learning disability, I have experienced firsthand the trials parents undergo in the world of childhood disabilities. Much of my training in this subject has been on the job, either as a clinician counseling a concerned parent over the intricacies of an Individualized Education Program, or as a frustrated parent myself wondering why no one can teach my son to read. In this chapter, I discuss the pediatrician's role in the team approach to the care of the child with a disability. My goal is to convey what your pediatrician can and cannot do for your child and for you.

MAJOR ROLES AND RESPONSIBILITIES OF PEDIATRICIANS

Despite the onslaught of managed care, threat of malpractice, and other medical horrors of the past decade, pediatrics is still an honored and satisfying profession. Pediatricians love kids, and enjoy working with their parents. In few other professions could one go to work wearing a Cat in the Hat tie, sit on the floor and play with toddlers (and get paid!). Even in the presence of terrible illness, there will always be reward in bringing comfort to children and their families.

Pediatricians are medical experts in development. It is the nature of their field. When development goes awry, it is their job to identify the problem, and if they cannot offer the solution themselves, to help guide their patients and their families through the process of diagnosis and therapy. They consider themselves patient advocates and allies (in contrast to managed care's attitude that doctors be technicians and gatekeepers). Pediatricians can handle many childhood problems themselves. Obviously, the more severe and/or complex the disorder, such as autism or cerebral palsy, the greater the need for other experts and ideas. Hence, the need for a team of experts.

There are limitations to pediatric expertise. Most of what pediatricians have been taught in school and specialty training involves physical disease and laboratory analysis. Unfortunately, in the field of some childhood disabilities, especially related to language and learning, pediatric training is still in the dark ages. Again, this is where the team approach is most useful. Educational experts, speech and language specialists, or physical and occupational therapists may become the primary caregivers for these children. The pediatrician may play more of an advisory role.

Pediatric Training

Following is a brief review of the training in the field of pediatrics. After completing college, a physician spends four years in medical school. The first two years involve mostly classroom study of the body and disease; the final two years are a classic apprenticeship on the wards of hospitals, in emergency rooms, or in physician's offices learning to relate to and care for patients. Greater emphasis has been placed on physician-patient communication in the past 10 years in medical schools. This area, however, is still deficient, as many readers may report in relating experiences with their doctors.

After medical school, there is a three-year training, or residency, in the specialty of pediatrics, usually housed in a pediatric hospital or the pediatric section of a general hospital. Here the apprenticeship continues. Much of this training is in illness related to children hospitalized with acute disease; that is, sick newborns, serious trauma, children with cancer or asthma, etc. Obviously, children with chronic or congenital disabilities, although occasionally admitted, are not a major focus of this kind of training. Following residency, the pediatrician may choose further training (fellowship) in a subspecialty field, such as gastroenterology or allergy. Outside of the fields directly related to disability, such as developmental pediatrics or neurology, most of this training does not touch on chronic disability. If a pediatrician does not choose to train in a subspecialty, he or she may then go into primary care practice.

So, if disabilities are an important part of pediatric practice, and relatively little is taught on this subject in training, where does a pediatrician learn about these children? On the job. Pediatric residents do not stop their education when they leave their residency or fellowship. Especially in the field of development, the pediatrician must maintain the desire to gain new knowledge in order to take better care of his or her patients. Physicians are required to take a set amount of continuing medical education, or CME, to maintain their medical licenses. This CME, whether in conferences, journal articles, or case reviews, is a valuable way of learning about development and disabilities. Discussion with specialists on the team, such as neurologists, psychologists, or speech-language pathologists, is another means of learning about the subject and current methods of diagnosis and therapy. Simply following several patients and their families through the maze of diagnosis, therapy and outcome is yet another method of learning. Patients and their families, even his own son, have taught this author more about this field than any residency ever could.

CONTRIBUTIONS OF MEDICINE TO INTERDISCIPLINARY PRACTICE

Pediatricians can feel quite a conflict when it comes to the team concept of care for children with disabilities. On the one hand, they are the primary medical caregiver, consoling and counseling parents, ordering tests and referrals, making plans, etc. On the other hand, they are frequently the one individual left out when it comes to meetings and long-range planning. They communicate with the other team members, but because of location, pediatricians in their offices and the team at a home, medical center, rehab facility, or school, they hear about plans and outcomes after the fact. It is important to understand that pediatricians do want to work within the team system, but efforts must be made by all, including the pediatrician and parent, to keep the doctor closely involved.

What follows is a review of how a pediatrician works, both individually and within the interdisciplinary team, to care for a child with chronic or congenital disabilities.

The Pediatrician's Job

So, what can your pediatrician do for your child and you when a problem is suspected? At the outset, the most important concept in the evaluation and therapy of a chronic disability is communication. Whether in person, by phone, by e-mail, or by letter, keeping in touch with patients during all phases of treatment is vital to a pediatrician. Most of the complaints concerning physicians involve some lack of communication. Explanations are incomplete, diagnostic tests are lost, misunderstandings arise; the end result is that everyone is unhappy. And most of all, lack of communication does not serve the patient's interest.

The hallmark of any physician-patient interaction is the medical history and physical exam. This step is no less important in chronic or congenital disabilities than in acute illnesses, as it is vital to determine whether medical disease is part (or the primary cause) of a child's problem. Again, communication between doctor, patient, and parents is key.

In reviewing the medical history of a child with disabilities, several issues are critical. What is the problem (i.e., symptoms)? What areas are involved: motor function, speech and language, reading, writing, paying attention, sitting still, emotional or physical outbursts, etc.? When was the problem first noticed (onset), and by whom? Were there any precipitating events, such as illness or emotional disturbance, or has it progressed gradually? Has there been evaluation or treatment done previously? By whom? And has anything helped?

Past medical history and family history can be quite important in the evaluation of a child with disabilities. Has the child had any chronic disease, especially affecting development or schooling? Was the child premature, or did the child have any birth defects? Was his or her development considered normal? And, if not, what were the problems, such as in motor, verbal, or social development? Were there any problems with hearing or speech (including chronic ear infections)? Did anyone else in the family, especially a parent or sibling, have such a problem? Do any childhood medical conditions "run" in the family, such as vision, hearing, or neurological problems?

The physical exam for a child with disabilities should involve a general exam with special emphasis on the specific areas of concern for that child; i.e., vision, hearing, neurologic, or other areas. For instance, abnormalities in physical appearance may suggest a genetic disorder, or findings on a neurologic exam may lead a physician to further explore a seizure or tic disorder.

Following the history taking and physical exam, the pediatrician may find it useful to discuss his or her findings with the parents and child, and to talk about the initial diagnoses. This gives the parents a chance to ask the doctor questions and provide further information that may not have come out before. Again and again, communication is vital.

Armed with some preliminary diagnoses, laboratory studies may be in order. Depending on the diagnostic possibilities, evaluation of blood chemistries, hormone function, or genetic material may be indicated. Radiological evaluation of the brain, brain wave testing (EEG), or specific testing of vision or hearing might be necessary. All of these tests are done with the cooperation and consent of the parents, and the pediatrician reviews all results with them. If referral to a pediatric specialist or allied health professional is needed, the pediatrician uses individuals he or she knows to be competent in their field and who will provide both the parents and the pediatrician with feedback in a timely fashion. The interdisciplinary team must work together if it is to help the patient. If insurance plans or the school system will become involved, the pediatrician's office provides parents with as much support and guidance as is possible to get them through the bureaucratic morass.

When a diagnosis is finally made and treatment is recommended, the pediatrician will again discuss this with the patient and family, even if another practitioner provides that diagnosis and treatment. Because of the relationship with the family, the pediatrician may be able to best interpret the medical jargon for the family. And they may be more at ease in asking him or her questions about their child's care. The pediatrician's role in the child's care does not end with a diagnosis. He or she must still be available to make further referrals, write prescriptions for chronic medications, write letters of necessity to insurance plans and school systems, and occasionally provide a shoulder for a parent or patient to cry on when things aren't going so well. Sometimes the pediatrician goes from being a counselor to a listener, and provides an even greater service.

The Pediatrician and the Team

As mentioned above, when a child with a chronic or congenital disability has problems which go beyond the range of the pediatrician to diagnose and/or manage, the pediatrician will make a referral to one or more members of the interdisciplinary team. The pediatrician's responsibility for the care of the child does not stop at this point. In fact, this responsibility becomes more significant as information from various sources must be collected and discussed with the family so that informed decisions can be made. The physician's management of his or her patient is now intertwined with the workings of the team.

The pediatrician, by dint of location, often feels left out of the team. However, this can be rectified by a concerted effort of the team members, the family, and the pediatrician to make sure they are kept constantly involved.

There is so much that the pediatrician can add to the team's functioning, both in the ongoing evaluation of the child and in the therapies that will be tried. The pediatrician knows the child's medical and developmental history better than anyone else involved, or, at the very least, has the best access to that information in the child's medical record. The pediatrician has examined the child, probably many times, and can best report on the medical and developmental problems affecting the whole child (not just the one organ system that a specialist is concerned with). The pediatrician has the best access to the list of medications the child has taken, the laboratory tests the child has undergone, and the specialist's notes for all the consultants the child has seen. They can provide ready access to this information and advice on caring for their patient to all members of the team. Finally, and perhaps most importantly, the pediatrician can act as the child's and family's representative to all the bureaucracy they face, including medical facilities (e.g., helping make appointments), schools (e.g., writing letters to school officials), and insurance companies (e.g., helping get claims paid).

Ultimately the participation of the pediatrician within the interdisciplinary team, although not always in the same room (or even the same city), is vital to the effective functioning of the team. And this, in turn, is in the best interest of the child and family.

THE ROLES PARENTS TYPICALLY PLAY IN THE OPTIMAL INTERDISCIPLINARY SERVICE PROVISION OF MEDICINE

It is obvious that if you are the parent or guardian of a child with a chronic or congenital disability and are reading this book, you are interested in participating in the team care for your child. Although the main focus of this chapter has been what a pediatrician can do for your child as an individual and as a member of the team, you, the parent, also have responsibility as part of the team.

In regard to the pediatrician, the parent is an important ally in the care of the child. There is no better source of medical information than the parent. Patient history, family history, hospital admissions, surgeries, consults, and allergies to medications are just some of the information a parent can collect, and then impart, to make the pediatrician's job easier. And parents do not have to memorize all this information. Just keeping this data in a file and bringing it in to the office for the child's visit will help enormously. Surely parents have already experienced the often painfully slow process of getting medical records from a former physician, or even worse, from a hospital. A record in the hand is worth fifty in some warehouse.

Learning about and cooperating with the pediatrician office's policies are other ways of helping the physician care for your child. Ask the office manager or head nurse how the office works. For example:

1. How do you make appointments?

This includes reserving sufficient time for an appointment for a child with a chronic illness. If you ever wondered, schedules are busiest for pediatricians during the winter (due to illness) and the summer (due to school and camp physicals).

2. How can you get copies of the medical record, which you may need for other interdisciplinary team members or outside agencies? Is there a charge for this (a common practice now)?

3. How can you get forms completed for schools, agencies and insurance companies?

Many forms need a physician's signature and/or some medical information, such as an immunization record. It is appropriate to expect a physician's office to complete these in a reasonable time. This is a nice way of saying, "don't wait until the last minute to get these to your doctor!"

4. How can you reach the physician for phone consultation?

Some offices have a call-in hour ("dialing for doctors"), whereas others use an advice nurse. It is likely that more parents call in to speak to the advice nurse than to speak to the pediatrician.

5. How can you get hold of a doctor in the office off-hours? What is the on-call system and who staffs it (if not your physician)?

6. What hospitals does your doctor use and/or recommend?

This is vital for a child with a chronic or congenital disability. Your physician should know best which institutions could handle the emergent care of such a child. The new "Doc in the Box" urgent care centers are not for everyone.

Again, the basic concept that should govern your interaction with your pediatrician is communication. You must choose the doctor you feel most comfortable with, someone willing to talk to you on a level you choose. Some doctors explain every last bit of information, asking for your input at every step, and taking pains to involve you in even the smallest of treatment decisions. Other doctors offer the more old fashioned "do this because I say so" technique of communication. And, of course, there are those who fall somewhere in between. Any one method is not necessarily the right one for every family. Just choose what works best for you. Don't be afraid to interview a doctor before choosing. And the best referrals to physicians always seem to come from other families who have used that physician.

In regards to the interdisciplinary team, the parent has the responsibility to make certain that all its members know who the child's primary care physician is. And they must continually remind them of this fact. This provides a vital link between the pediatrician and other team members. Make certain that all consultants' notes on evaluation and therapy will be sent to your pediatrician. By so doing, both you and the pediatrician have ready access to them. Even better, your pediatrician can interpret them for you and help you decide what the next steps in evaluation or therapy should be. Finally, make certain that you have a pediatrician who is willing to communicate with the other members of the team. A very busy doctor cannot drop what he or she is doing and accept calls from or meet with the team at any given moment. However, a physician must be flexible. Calls from team members must be returned in a timely fashion and input from the pediatrician, even if in a letter or over the phone, must be given to the team.

My experience with my own son's learning disability has given me a greater appreciation for what parents go through in the world of chronic childhood disability. I, too, have sat through the hours of psychological testing and on the phone with the insurance company afterward, trying to convince them that his testing was medically necessary. I, too, have been frustrated by the endless conferences with specialists and the even more tedious school meetings. I have seen where the interdisciplinary team works and where it breaks down. As I've said repeatedly, communication is the key.

What can your pediatrician do for your child and you? Give explanations that you can understand. Discuss all treatment options and the best people or institutions to carry out that treatment. Work closely with other members of the team. Be honest, whether the news is good or bad. And above all, be there when you need them.

What can you do for your pediatrician? Schedule well ahead for conferences and physical exams, allowing for enough time to discuss problems and plans. Make certain that all necessary forms, referrals, prescriptions, and other paperwork are requested in a timely fashion. Keep them up to date on recommendations and treatments by other practitioners. And remember that your pediatrician is one of your child's most important allies in the complicated world of childhood disabilities.

TYPICAL PARENT QUESTIONS/COMMENTS FOR PEDIATRICIANS

I'd like for my pediatrician to attend school IEP meetings and other meetings where he could provide valuable insight. Is this too much to ask?

Yes, it is too much to expect your pediatrician to attend the IEP meetings. But that does not relinquish your pediatrician from the responsibility of supporting your child and you through this difficult process.

For the uninitiated, the school IEP (Individualized Educational Program) meetings are held to determine the school's program for your child with special needs. In some areas, these are known as ARD (Admission, Review, and Discharge) meetings. Generally, members of the school team, which may include teachers, speech-language pathologists, reading specialists, occupational therapists, psychologists, and/or an administrator, meet with the parents to see what needs must be met for the child within the school system. Unfortunately, in this day of restricted budgets, limiting, not broadening, services to a child may be one of the goals of these meetings. To make matters worse, these meetings can be quite intimidating to a parent with little background in the educational system and knowledge of the technical language. I have sat through such sessions for my son, and even with extensive pediatric training, I was frequently lost ("When are they going to get to the part about teaching him how to read?" I kept wondering). Therefore, it would certainly be nice to have an expert ally in the room with you at the meeting.

The pediatrician should play an important part in the patient's IEP process. Usually, the pediatrician schedules conferences with the parents prior to the IEP meeting to go over the child's needs. These conferences are optimal usually at the end of the day when the pediatrician's full attention can be devoted to the problem. In addition, the pediatrician may prepare a letter detailing what he or she feels is vital for the child's education. If necessary, the pediatrician can speak with school personnel concerning the child, and voice opinions (over the phone or in writing) concerning the resulting IEP. Finally, and perhaps most importantly, the pediatrician helps the parents in choosing the right educational consultant to advise and accompany them to the meeting. Depending on the child's disability, the consultant may be an educational specialist, a psychologist, or a language specialist, who has experience with the convoluted IEP process. More than the pediatrician, they can represent the child's interests in an arena they understand.

One final note. These meetings always occur during school hours, and could take two to three hours out of a pediatrician's already busy day. In this era of managed care, the primary care pediatrician is rarely paid for this service. Think of what a lawyer would charge for a two-hour conference with a client. It just is not feasible for your doctor, with patients clamoring for appointments, referrals, prescription refills, etc., to take that time out of the office.

I have experienced physicians who are quick to prescribe medication for children with autism. I believe redirection is the key to more appropriate behaviors. What is your view about medicating persons with autism who exhibit behavioral excesses?

Despite extensive research, autism remains a complex and little understood disorder. To confuse the matter, it has been grouped with other developmental disorders under the cryptic diagnosis of Pervasive Developmental Disorder, or PDD. The hallmarks of autistic behavior are deficits in social interaction, language, communication, and play, and a narrowed range of interests and activities. Children with autism may have marked behavioral abnormalities, including problems with attention, aggressiveness, perseveration, anxiety, and destructiveness.

This question addresses whether medication or redirection (i.e., a form of behavior therapy) is more effective in the treatment of an autistic child. Unfortunately, there is no treatment yet discovered which will cure autism. Certainly, therapies aimed at resolving the behavioral and communication problems are the most helpful interventions presently available. Some medications have been quite helpful in controlling abnormalities such as anxiety and impulsiveness in many children with autism. Alternatively, a highly-structured environment using one-on-one interaction with the child is a behavioral method that has shown benefit. The treatment plan needs to be individualized for the specific needs of each child with autism. A mixture of behavioral techniques and medication may be best for some children.

Just because the child's ability to communicate is impaired does not mean that our ability to communicate as parent and physician should likewise be affected. Prescribing a medication to treat a behavior without the consent or understanding of a parent is unwise and doomed to failure. Conversely, the parent trying inappropriate behavioral techniques without the advice and support of the medical/educational team will meet with an equally bad result. The treatment plan for a child with autism needs to be discussed among and agreed to by the parents, the treating physician, and the other specialists and educators involved in the care of the child. The plan may need to be tailored to the different situations the child encounters. Redirection may work in the less stressful milieu of home while medication might be necessary at school.

The pediatrician should sit down and discuss all treatment options with the parents, pros and cons, in order to come to an agreement on what is best for the child. A pediatrician can do this even if, as is frequently the case, he or she is not the individual recommending a specific medicine or behavior therapy. It is the family and the pediatrician who have the best interests of the child at heart.

How can professionals be encouraged to be patient with parents given all that comes along with parenting a child with special needs? It is not easy to accept that my child is not as perfect as I see him.

More time is spent in medical school on diagnosing and treating medical illness than on communication skills. Doctors and other medical professionals have spent years of their lives learning the intricacies of complex medical disorders and what to do for them. But, as is painfully obvious to many parents of children with disabilities, a professional's ability to listen to the patient and family, and then communicate, is usually lacking. In truth, the pressures of managed care and increased workloads do not always allow time to discuss both family and physician concerns in a relaxed fashion. It is hard to fully discuss the issues when there are other patients to see and other families to counsel. However, for the good of the child, this must somehow happen.

No matter what their disability, all parents view their children as special and, in their own way, perfect. It is not easy for the parent, nor, in truth, is it easy for the doctor to bring up the poor growth, painfully slow development or difficult behavior that many of these children with disabilities have. However, these are the things parents and pediatricians must discuss, as it is the child, not themselves, they are trying to help. The pediatrician can try to block out sufficient time for these conferences (or schedule them toward the end of the day) so as to minimize interruptions. It is good for the pediatrician to give all the news, good or bad, as he or she sees it and then allow time for discussion and counseling. The pediatrician must continually assess the parents' understanding of diagnoses and treatment plans. They must work together. In doing this, a pediatrician will have his or her share of making parents cry over the years with answers they didn't want to hear.

Seek out those professionals who are willing to talk, to take the time to communicate. Whether good news or bad, your child will be best served by such a caregiver.

Editors' Note:
   We wish every physician could read this chapter, particularly the words "sometimes I go from being a counselor to a listener" and "...be there when you need them."

In Jane Schulz's words:

   Although he had all the stigmata of Down syndrome, Billy was 18 months old before we had a diagnosis. Two pediatricians had told us to "just give him time." The third pediatrician gave us the correct diagnosis, after consulting with his partner, with tears running down his face. This expression of empathy was the dearest thing I had ever seen.
   I realize that physicians' training is more thorough now than when Billy was born. However, if parents do not receive satisfactory answers to their questions, they should go elsewhere. We are advised not "to shop around," but in such an important event, it is foolish not to seek more than one opinion.
   Honesty is critical at the time of diagnosis. Even when the news is not good, it is better than uncertainty.

Chapter 4

NUTRITION

SARAH MCCAMMAN AND JANE RUES

MAJOR RESPONSIBILITIES AND ROLES OF NUTRITIONISTS

The goals of pediatric nutrition are to improve children's nutrition and growth, prevent retardation or further disability, help children experience fewer illnesses, improve performance in home and educational settings, and provide education and support to the child and caregivers. In order for nutrition programs to accomplish these goals, they must be provided by qualified professionals who are able to relate the assessment of dietary intake with a health history, physical examination, laboratory findings and the child's clinical status to formulate recommendations regarding diet, behavioral issues, and feeding concerns. A comprehensive interview and the ability to integrate information from a variety of disciplines are key skills necessary to develop and implement a nutrition plan. Competence to teach the skills necessary to make changes in diet and lifestyle is also a critical skill for a nutritionist.

A registered dietician has a bachelor's degree, has passed a national registration examination, and in many states must be licensed to practice. Unfortunately, not all those who call themselves nutritionists have completed this rigorous licensing process. Some individuals calling themselves nutritionists will have little or no formal education in nutrition principles or in health issues of children. When seeking help for the complex nutrition concerns that children with special health care needs present, choose a professional with specialized advanced training in the field of nutrition. Nutrition-related concerns commonly encountered in this population include: alterations in growth, possible nutrient deficiencies, eating/feeding issues, constipation, drug-nutrient interactions, and assessment of alternative therapies. The expertise of the nutritionist is an essential component of health care for children who are at increased nutritional risk.

Common Problems

One of the most common nutrition challenges encountered in children with developmental disabilities is the assessment of growth, including both weight gain and linear growth. Energy balance concerns are common and include issues related to failure to thrive, obesity, and slower than usual growth in height. Energy needs of children with special health care concerns are highly variable requiring an individualized assessment. For example, children with Down syndrome, Prader-Willi syndrome, Lawrence-Moon-Beidel syndrome, or spina bifida generally have lower energy levels than children who are typically developing; their growth rate is slower and thus these youngsters have increased risk of being overweight. In contrast, children with cerebral palsy, bronchopulmonary dysplasia, or congenital heart disease tend to need more calories than the child who is typically developing; they can be underweight for their height and occasionally suffer from severe malnutrition manifested by no weight gain or weight loss and stunted linear growth.

Assessing linear growth of youngsters with special health care needs can be challenging. For children with physical attributes that make standing difficult (spina bifida, scoliosis, cerebral palsy), estimations of height are based on arm span, sitting height, knee height or other techniques that compensate for the disability. Using one of these alternative methods allows the nutrition professional to obtain serial length/height-related data and monitor linear growth in addition to weight gain.

A lower than optimal intake of one or more nutrients is a common finding among children who have a limited food intake. A limited food intake can be due to oral motor impairments, frequent illness, reduced energy needs, side effects from medications, or dietary restrictions. Education and counseling by a nutrition professional can identify this problem early, before it leads to malnutrition.

Some children with special health care needs require placement of a nasogastric or gastrostomy tube because of an inability to consume adequate calories orally. Frequently, the tube feeding is temporary and a return to at least partial oral feeds can be achieved. The nutritionist is valuable in helping to determine the type, amount, and timing of tube feedings, as well as the composition and volume of foods to be offered to maintain good nutritional status during the transition from tube to oral feeds.

Another common nutrition-related issue for children with special health care needs is constipation. Constipation can result from a low fiber diet, medications, poor fluid intake, decreased physical activity, and high or low muscle tone. The usual recommendations by nutritionists are to increase fluid, dietary fiber, and daily exercise. Strategies for how to best incorporate these recommendations in situations where children have oral motor difficulties, physical limitations, or restricted food choices necessitate working closely with the child and family to individualize the nutrition plan.

Children with special health care needs may also require long-term use of a number of medications. Drug therapy can interfere with nutrient metabolism, and may produce nutrition-related side effects such as altered growth, increased nutrient needs, bone demineralization, obesity, loss of appetite, constipation, nausea, vomiting, or gastric distress. The nutritionist can provide assistance with the timing of meals and medications, advice on the use of vitamin and mineral supplements, and suggest dietary changes to prevent or reduce the nutrition-related side-effects.

Nutrition problems encountered in children with special health care needs tend to be multiple, complex, and overlapping. The earlier the problem is identified, the less severe the effects and the greater the likelihood of successful treatment. The purpose of nutrition screening is to identify children with an existing nutrition concern or a potential problem. Because children with special health care needs are at considerable risk for nutrition-related problems, it is important that routine nutrition screening be provided. A screening can be accomplished by a variety of individuals including paraprofessionals, teachers, physicians' assistants, or other health care providers. When a child is identified as having one or more nutritional risk factors he or she needs to be referred for a nutrition assessment.

A nutrition professional should perform the nutrition assessment. A nutrition assessment is the collection and evaluation of data in five categories: body measurements, clinical status, biochemical data, dietary intake, development of feeding skill and behaviors around mealtimes. If the assessment confirms the existence of a nutrition problem, intervention should be provided by a nutritionist that may include consultation with professionals from a variety of disciplines.

CONTRIBUTIONS OF NUTRITION TO
INTERDISCIPLINARY PRACTICE

Nutritional issues are not isolated, but are one aspect to be considered in the child's overall development. The child's health, social, motor, communication, and cognitive skills are affected by his or her nutritional status.

The significance of nutritional information is evidenced by the representation of nutritionists on interdisciplinary teams developed to meet the needs of children with special health care needs. Children with cerebral palsy, cleft palate, spina bifida, inborn errors of metabolism (e.g., PKU), etc., are often served by professionals from a variety of disciplines. The composition of the team is dictated by diagnostic and treatment characteristics of a particular population of children. Although the composition changes are based on the diagnosis, nutrition is generally a constant across pediatric interdisciplinary teams.

The availability and visibility of the nutritionist as a team member has increased in the past 10 to 15 years. This is a result of several factors, notably awareness of the prevalence of pediatric nutritional disorders and of the importance of nutrition to early development. A number of early studies documented that a large percentage of children with developmental disabilities received inadequate nutrition for growth and development (Palmer, 1978; Peaks & Lamb, 1951). A more recent survey of over 2,000 special education students suggested that 37 percent of the children needed special foods or diets and 32 percent required special feeding procedures (i.e., tube feeding, modified feeding equipment, or supervision at mealtime) (Horsley, 1988). A recent review of the health records of 50 students with profound disabilities documented that 47 percent of the students had growth retardation with weight-for-height below the fifth percentile (Ault, Guy, Rues, Noto, & Guess, 1994). Today most professionals and the general public know the basics of nutrition; this increase in awareness has resulted in an appreciation for the contribution nutrition makes to health and development.

Team members look to the nutrition professional for assistance with the complex problems that are encountered in the feeding/eating process. Analysis of the nutritional value of what the child is eating and drinking and the impact of diet on growth and health are accomplished competently and efficiently by the pediatric nutritionist. The team, which includes the family, is also aware that a prerequisite or antecedent to alert responsive behavior and good health is adequate nutrition. From a developmental point of view, an inadequately nourished child may be physiologically compromised as he or she attempts to interact with persons or materials in the environment. Characteristics of students receiving inadequate nutrition include lethargy, easily decreased levels of energy or stamina, and poor attention span. The child with a chronic illness or developmental disability will benefit more from the recommended interventions if the child is alert and responsive to the environment.

The nutrition professional, working with the team, screens, evaluates, and provides follow-up. Team members are often trained to gather preliminary data in one or more of the following categories: body measurements, clinical status, biochemical information, dietary intake, socioeconomic situation, development of feeding skills, and behavioral issues related to the feeding situation. Table 4-1 provides a Screening Checklist of common problems developed to assist other team members in the screening process.

Table 4-1
SCREENING CHECKLIST

		YES	NO
1.	Underweight (Wt/Ht <5%)	____	____
2.	Overweight (Wt/Ht >95%)	____	____
3.	No weight gain in one month (B-12 months)	____	____
4.	No weight gain in three months (1- 2 years)	____	____
5.	Average meal exceeds 30-40 minutes	____	____
6.	Average meal is less than 10 minutes	____	____
7.	Difficulty swallowing or sucking	____	____
8.	Excessive crying, whining, or signs of discomfort during and/or after a meal	____	____
9.	Frequent gagging, coughing, or choking	____	____
10.	Difficult to position for feeding	____	____
11.	Exclusive breast or formula fed at 9-10 months	____	____
12.	Not on table food at 16 months	____	____
13.	Refusal to eat one food group	____	____
14.	Primarily on gavage feedings	____	____

This checklist can be used to routinely screen all children and then serve as referral criteria to a nutritionist and/or a feeding team. The ultimate goal of screening is to provide early nutrition intervention or anticipatory guidance for those at risk for nutrition problems. Nutritional assessment findings, covered earlier in this chapter, must be translated into realistic and specific recommendations that are integrated with the team's recommendations and prioritized to meet the needs of the child and family.

Nutritional Interventions

Nutritional issues and needs are dynamic and changing. An essential aspect of intervention is follow-up which may include ongoing monitoring, reevaluation, and program modification.

The role of follow-up is critical to the youngster with a chronic illness and/or developmental disability. The efficacy of the recommended nutritional intervention will be evidenced by improved growth and health but may also be reflected in the child's improved performance in other developmental areas. Intervention strategies for students whose health is compromised require that the team consider a range and sequence of alternatives. For example, in the case of a chronically, severely undernourished child, the first priority is to increase caloric intake to acceptable levels. The alternatives may include: (1) increasing caloric density of oral feeds and increasing the number of meals throughout the day or (2) combining oral feeds with tube feeding. The collaborative plan may involve implementation of the first intervention with monitoring that assesses its effect on health, growth, and development. The monitoring phase allows for an analysis of the data by the family, health and/or educational providers to determine the direction and magnitude of the change and whether additional intervention or continued monitoring is indicated. The occupational and physical therapist and early childhood teacher may report an increase in responsiveness and tolerance for activity which may be a function of increased caloric and nutrient consumption. Clearly, the nutritionist's membership on the interdisciplinary team is critical to the child and family; he or she must be an effective communicator and collaborator with the immediate team and the community based team.

Nutritionists As Collaborative Team Members

Collaboration among the child's family, diagnostic team, and community-based team is essential. When the roles of various team members are respected, success in nutritional management of children with specific needs can be assured.

The nutritionist relies on the skills of the other team members and collaboration with these professionals to gather information important to the process of clinical problem solving. This is perhaps best exemplified by the issues surrounding feeding, a major challenge for many children with special health care needs. Feeding issues encompass personal mealtime characteristics, food choices, oral-motor development, eating/feeding skills, behaviors around mealtime, and use of tube feedings. Limited amounts of food, restricted varieties of food, and/or behavioral problems around mealtime such as tantrums, food refusal, or resistance to texture change, will affect the caloric and nutritional adequacy of the child's diet. Children who have difficulty sucking or swallowing or who frequently gag, choke, cough, cry, whine, or show signs of discomfort such as vomiting or cramping are also at risk for inadequate intake and poor growth. These characteristics may be observed in children who are orally fed, gastrostomy fed, or a combination of the two (Ault, Guy, & Rues, 1992; McCamman & Rues, 1990). Many of these feeding difficulties are a result of neuromuscular dysfunction, obstructive lesions, or past unpleasant experiences associated with the mouth or feeding. The problems are complex, often long-standing, and physically and emotionally draining for the family and clearly exemplify the need for collaboration among the interdisciplinary team members.

The social worker provides data regarding family needs and resources; the speech-language pathologist and occupational and physical therapists examine the oral-motor and motor skills and provide important information about positioning and feeding techniques; the speech-language pathologist assists in the analysis of swallowing; and the nurse and/or physician inform the team of the natural history of the child's diagnosis and potential indications or contraindications of various recommendations. These interactions are crucial and enhance the capacity for the provision of comprehensive services. This openness to collaboration in clinical problem solving provides a context for the team to prioritize the recommendations.

Collaboration provides a vehicle for organizing and sharing information with a community-based team who may be responsible for implementation of team recommendations. The ability of the diagnostic team to identify professionals within the family's community and to train these individuals to carry out the intervention program will impact the ease with which the goals are achieved. Careful monitoring and follow-up by nutrition and other team members are key to maintaining the family and professionals' commitment to the program. The utilization of technology (e.g., electronic mail) provides an accessible and efficient way to quickly communicate progress and/or problems with recommended interventions. Sequential video tapes of the child during the feeding process provides the entire team, diagnostic and community-based, with an important chronology of the treatment program and also becomes a method to capture and share the child's performance for mutual and continued problem solving.

THE ROLES PARENTS TYPICALLY PLAY IN THE OPTIMAL INTERDISCIPLINARY SERVICE PROVISION OF NUTRITION

Parents are the real experts on their child; they are experts about the child's likes, dislikes, strengths and needs. Each family has unique approaches to foods, mealtimes, and activities around food. Values and beliefs around foods and eating must be respected and integrated into the child's program.

Professionals vary in the roles they expect families to play; families vary in the roles they assume. This can range from the family being viewed as part of the child's problem to that of a collaborator, critical to team function. Families can no longer be viewed as passive and grateful recipients of professional information, nor may they choose the role of a fully functioning team member who actively participates in all decisions. The family's role with the team will evolve. Regardless of their level of involvement, their commitment must be acknowledged through respect and regard for the information they provide. Clearly no one role can fit all families; nor do we limit our view of the family to the traditional mother-child dyad—rather, we consider the family as a unit. Failure to include and consider all family members may engender feelings of shame, incompetence, and exclusion. It may foster distance from the child with a disability, i.e., family members who are not viewed as resources may begin to question their competence in other issues related to family functioning.

The family's motivation, skill and knowledge are available when they are equal and full partners with other team members. This collaboration is mutually beneficial; it brings multiple perspectives and resources otherwise unavailable. The role of collaborator is essential to maximize the resources necessary to provide the most successful experiences for a child with a disability.

The benefits of collaboration are easily seen in the team work necessary to assess the complex problems of youngsters with feeding concerns. The family participates by identifying problems, providing background information, prioritizing issues, helping to develop strategies, practicing interventions, and providing feedback on the feasibility of carrying out the recommendations and the success of the interventions. Parents often provide important background information by recording the foods and fluids eaten by the child each day in a food record. This record is analyzed by the nutritionist. The record provides opportunities to discuss family traditions around food, cultural attitudes about food, eating patterns, as well as providing the team with data on the nutrient intake. These cultural traditions, once identified, are acknowledged and honored as the recommendations are developed.

Parents are also critical in establishing priorities for the team. For example, a youngster with spina bifida may present with obesity, constipation, and oral sensitivity to textured food. The family may choose to work on increasing texture and fiber in the diet to relieve the constipation while not immediately addressing the issue of obesity. Maximizing flexibility and promoting choices are important when developing treatment strategies. Each family is different and has its own characteristics, styles of interactions, and rituals regarding food. It is essential that families feel free to express themselves openly.

If caregivers are expected to integrate recommendations into their daily activities, their input on what is reasonable regarding frequency and intensity is imperative. Their sense of ownership and competence must be maintained and nurtured by professionals, not threatened. The opportunity to practice the interventions with feedback from the professionals is essential to building confidence and competence in caring for their child. Mealtime can be used to increase the skill level of parents while simultaneously identifying with the parent how their infant communicates his or her preferences, pleasure, joy, and displeasure. Enhancing quality of parent-infant interactions requires that these cues be identified and responded to if mealtime is to become a setting for successful reciprocal communication between parent and child.

Supporting parents in making decisions about using alternative, nonstandard therapies is a growing responsibility of the nutritionist. Today, more and more Americans are focusing on the effects of nutrition and diet on health which have contributed to a significant number of families exploring nontraditional therapies. The support, information, and hope of improvement promised by proponents of controversial therapies may be attractive to families, especially when standard treatments can be difficult to access, confusing, costly, and time consuming. Parents often feel excluded from important treatment decisions and feel frustrated and overwhelmed by multiple and conflicting treatment recommendations. Nutrition professionals have a responsibility to remain actively involved and available to parents to openly discuss any treatment that they may choose.

Look Again

This first vignette presents a youngster and his mother's interaction with a feeding team over a period of 10 years. Martin P. had been followed since birth by an interdisciplinary diagnostic and feeding team located in a major tertiary medical center. In addition, the youngster had received educational services through a transdisciplinary preschool program located within the medical center. Martin, a child with severe and multiple handicaps, and his single mother were well-known to members of the team. A variety of feeding related interventions had been implemented over the years by both the preschool staff and his mother; these interventions had resulted in only varying degrees of success as this youngster continued to present with weight-for-height below the 5th percentile. His mother met with team members formally and informally during the preschool years and spoke of her frustration with the amount of time spent daily feeding her son with "so little to show for it." The team attempted to respond to the mother's requests, but the solutions were never entirely successful. When Martin reached school age, he transferred to the public school and the majority of his services were provided through the school district.

The team was contacted periodically by either the school or Martin's mother with concerns regarding feeding that impacted his growth and health. Again the team revisited its earlier recommendations and efforts were renewed to increase the caloric and nutritional composition of Martin's meals, while continuing to work on his oral-motor skills.

When Martin was 12 years of age, his mother made an appointment with the feeding team and requested the team to look at her son with "fresh eyes," i.e., not to be influenced by his long history, but rather look at this 12-year-old boy who weighed only 45 pounds. This had the desired effect on the entire team and resulted in a radically different approach to this youngster's management. A gastrostomy tube was recommended to meet his nutritional needs and four weeks after the tube was placed Martin had gained seven pounds. In addition to the very important weight gain, his health improved (skin breakdown healed quickly) and he experienced increased levels of alertness. Although his mother continued to offer preferred foods orally, she was no longer spending the majority of her evening hours trying unsuccessfully to feed him orally.

This mother's perseverance, focus, and communication skills demanded that the team look again at this child.

Goal Identification

John M. is a four-month-old who has Cornelia de Lange syndrome and a cleft palate. His mother requested a nutrition consultation while in the Cleft Palate Clinic because she wanted to make sure his nutritional needs were being met from the breast milk she was pumping and feeding. She also wanted to know how to pump more milk in a shorter period of time and, if possible, to put him to the breast and avoid the breast pumping. She arrived in the nutrition suite with John, her husband, and their four other youngsters. During the interview it became obvious that John's level of care was having a tremendous impact on the entire family. Mrs. M. spends about four to six hours per day pumping breast milk and feeding her son. She pumps her breasts five to six times per day and feeds John every three to four hours for approximately 40 minutes. John is an irritable infant, difficult to console, who spits up frequently.

His weight gain is marginal, slightly below the 5th percentile for weight for age; he is at the 5th percentile for height for age and at the 10th percentile weight for height. Mrs. M. expressed the concern that her other children were breastfed for a year and she believes John deserves the same. She is worried that he will not tolerate infant formula since he already is a difficult to feed youngster and seems to be only marginally tolerating breast milk. She is not sure he will get the benefits from breast milk if any formula is added. She also expressed concern that her other children have been basically "on their own" since John was born and they are beginning to have some problems in school and at home. Mr. M. stated that they are unable to continue the intense level of care that John requires.

After an extensive interview, the following issues were identified by members of the health care team working with John. Did his symptoms of irritability, arching, and spitting symptoms suggest gastroesophageal reflux? What were techniques to enhance milk flow during pumping? Was John being fed with the most efficient feeding device? What would it take to make feeding from the breast an option? Was a nasogastric tube an option for short-term relief? What were some parent-to-parent resources for this family?

With family participation, each issue was openly and fully discussed with the appropriate professional. Mrs. M. decided that the steps necessary to help John feed directly from the breast (repeated visits to the dentist for the fitting of an obturator) were not feasible given the travel required and the additional stress this would place on the family. A more appropriate bottle and nipple were recommended that would decrease the amount of time necessary to feed John. An electric pump was rented, reducing by half the amount of time it took to pump the same amount of milk. She was reassured that the addition of infant formula as a supplement would not interfere with the benefits John was receiving from the breast milk. The total amount of fluids offered was then increased through a combination of breast milk and formula to promote weight gain. The irritability, arching, and spitting were identified as reflux esophagitis and medication to normalize motility and decrease the acid production in his stomach were prescribed. Phone numbers were given for local parent-to-parent support groups as well as the national support group for families with youngsters with Cornelia de Lange syndrome.

Follow-up by phone to monitor feeding behavior, success with the new pump, weight gain, and tolerance of the medications occurred weekly. John quickly became less fussy and more easily consoled. Mrs. M. was able to decrease the amount of time she spent pumping and feeding. Within a month, she had increased the amount of formula offered to meet his increasing calorie level. His weight gain was adequate. The family opted not to become involved with any support groups because it was "too depressing to hear about so many youngsters with so many problems."

John, his family, and the professionals exemplify a true team. They treated each other with mutual respect and trust, acknowledging the experience and knowledge that each brought to the relationship. Open communication existed and all were free to share and question; they also recognized that negotiation and commitment were essential to successful team collaboration and problem solving.

TYPICAL PARENT QUESTIONS/COMMENTS FOR NUTRITIONISTS

Why is it so difficult to get people to operate as a team? I'm frustrated because I get so many contradictory opinions and often feel like the "middle man" for professionals who don't work together. Do you have suggestions?

Not all roles that families have are welcome or justified. Unfortunately, parents sometimes find themselves with professionals who do not work together as a team, who do not meet their needs, and they are then forced to assume the role of a "middle-man" coordinating communication among disparate team members. These communication mismatches occur for a variety of reasons: lack of understanding and trust among team members, lack of a common goal, and/or lack of a common language to communicate that goal.

Experts on team formation and structure acknowledge that the evolution of a team is more successful if the group has a common context or goal that focuses the individual members (e.g., a family-focus). Team members who represent different disciplines, different theoretical perspectives, and different levels of educational preparation require a central unifying context to assist and motivate them to reconcile these other perceived differences. Although team relationships are formed over time, this formation is rarely smooth and some teams self-destruct early in the process. Characteristics of successful teams include a defined and unifying philosophy, a commitment to working through the inevitable personality issues, a common language and a comprehensive system of evaluation. Evaluation should be continuous and provide the team with information regarding their effectiveness, efficiency and responsiveness to families and children. Ongoing feedback of this nature maintains integrity, avoids complacency, and expedites a proactive stance. Teams are also constantly changing; as members come and go the dynamics of the team are altered, requiring adaptation and accommodation of the remaining members. This, then, is the situation for families and we hope an understanding of this process will assist families as they negotiate with teams. Strategies families have used to enhance communication among team members will now be shared.

An important first step is the family's ability to identify, articulate, and prioritize the child's problem(s) for the team. The use of the family's "own words" creates a common language for the team; likewise, the family's priorities assist the team in establishing common goals. Shared responsibility occurs as the team is able to focus on the issues and recognize that the expertise of the entire group, including the family, is critical to successful problem solving. Some families have found it useful to identify or recruit an ally to the team. Since families prefer frequent and informal communication on issues involving their children (Turnbull & Turnbull, 1997), these individuals can help advocate for team meetings, more frequent and varied communication, including written communication, (e.g., handbooks, handouts, newsletters, dialogue journals, letters, and report cards). Telephone contact is also convenient and effective. The frequency of telephones in the American home (94 percent) is higher than our literacy rate. With so many homes and offices having answering machines, contacting each other in this manner has become quite popular. Other forms of technology (i.e., e-mail, video, microrecorders) are also becoming more common and should be utilized when available to increase timely information flow among team members.

There are also many forms of face-to-face contact. Successful meetings require planning and follow-up to be most effective. Planning the agenda, submitting questions ahead of time, arranging the environment, recording the proceedings, and evaluating the outcomes are some of the tasks necessary to assure best outcome. Although unplanned meetings or dropping by a classroom before school do provide one-to-one contact, these interactions rarely provide satisfactory communication among a group of people.

Teamwork is an event requiring shared responsibility, common language, and common goals. The family's gentle insistence on clarity and consensus among team members will solidify and define their role and create a milieu for communication.

Dr. Schulz's Response:

When Billy was a teenager, we moved to a small town. He began experiencing severe abdominal pains and we took him to a family physician, who referred him to a surgeon. The surgeon diagnosed the problem as a hernia, and set up a date for surgery.

I wasn't satisfied with this diagnosis, and called a trusted friend who is a nurse. She suggested that I take Billy to a pediatrician, someone she had good experience with. The pediatrician said, "Let's look at other possibilities. We know that people with Down syndrome tend to be constipated, so let's try that first." A laxative brought instant relief, and attention to diet contributed to solution of the problem. This avoided surgery, which would not have solved the problem anyway.

This experience suggests several approaches to me. First, sometimes parents have to be aggressive—if results do not please you, act on your own. Second, trust your own instincts. If a professional suggests something that does not feel right to you, question it or investigate other sources. Third, you may find that pediatricians will have suggestions applicable to your adult family member who has a disability. I continued taking Billy to this particular pediatrician until I found someone in my community who was knowledgeable about Down syndrome.

What kind of nutritional therapy is available for persons with autism? What does the literature say about its effectiveness?

In a recent survey of parents with children who were diagnosed with autism, about half had tried at least one alternative therapy (Nickle, 1996). These therapies are generally categorized as nutritional or behavioral. Of the nutritional therapies available, the most popular is supplementation with vitamin B6 and magnesium. Although there are over 50 papers in the literature discussing the effects of supplements on children with autism, it is difficult at this time to identify a causal relationship between supplementation and improved outcome (Pfeiffer, Norton, Nelson, & Shott, 1995). While some studies suggest that children and adults with autism benefit from large daily doses of supplements, virtually all of these reports have design flaws that make it impossible to draw any valid conclusions. Because no consistent and positive effect can be shown from large doses of vitamins and minerals and a very real danger of serious side effects exists, it is recommended that if a family chooses to give supplements, they do so under the guidance of a physician and nutritionist. Clear treatment objectives and pre/post supplement assessment of these objectives to document any response to therapy will ensure that the health of the child is not compromised.

Can medications cause weight gain? If so what can be done to manage the weight gain given the need for the medication?

Yes, medication can cause individuals to gain weight. Specific, common offenders include steroids and valporic acid. Prevention of undesirable weight gain is always easier than losing weight and should begin with education. Certain drugs may increase desire for sweets and other foods; thus high calorie foods and beverages, should be restricted. While using the drug, intake of low calorie foods, beverages and snacks is encouraged; additionally, incorporation of high-fiber foods and snacks into the diet may contribute to early satiety. An emphasis on increased physical activity may also help with weight maintenance. If weight gain is one of the side effects commonly found with a medication then it is recommended that the individual have frequent weight checks to allow a quick reversal of small weight gain. Finally, the individual should be informed that drug-related food cravings may diminish and weight may be lost after drug discontinuation.

As a professional, how do you find out information about rare disorders?

Over the last few years the Internet has dramatically changed the availability of information about rare disorders. Extensive and comprehensive information is now easily available to all interested individuals through a number of sites that specialize in rare disorders. A good place to get started is the Office of Rare Diseases at the National Institutes of Health. Another, the National Organization for Rare Disorders, is a federation of voluntary health organizations dedicated to helping people with rare "orphan" diseases. Additionally, the families of individuals with rare disorders have a wealth of knowledge about their individual family member as well as generalities about the disorder, support groups, and the names of professionals who have experience in this disorder. The family is always the expert on their family member.

What do you do to find out the individual needs of the children you see and their families?

The process of identifying these concerns and priorities can begin with a written questionnaire to be completed and returned by the family before the first visit. The process of completing this intake information may help the family articulate their needs for the nutritionist. This preliminary information can help prepare the professional for the first face-to-face contact with the family. During the initial interview, the family should be asked directly about their concerns and what they want to get out of the visit. Open and honest communication with attention to both verbal and nonverbal communication will result in an interaction that addresses the needs of the child and family and that is personally and professionally satisfying for the professional.

Is there truth to the proposed relationship between hyperactivity and various foods? If so, what should I eliminate from my son's diet?

A number of dietary factors have been proposed as causes for hyperactivity. These include sugar, food additives, and allergens. A recent analysis of 23 studies found no effect of sugar (mainly sucrose) on children's behavior and cognition. In other words, sugar did not make most children "hyper." It is possible that a small subset of children do increase their activity level in response to sugar consumption; however, the small number of reliable studies performed to date do not address this issue for individual children. The question remains, why do the results of well-controlled studies differ so much from the impressions of parents? We know that parents are excellent and reliable observers of behavior. It is hypothesized that excited states in children are common at birthday parties, Halloween, and other events where sugar is consumed. The increased activity associated with these occasions may be mistakenly correlated with sugar consumption.

Children with food allergies may exhibit irritability, fatigue, and difficulty with concentration. If a child is suspected of having a food allergy a physician should be consulted for a diagnosis. A consultation with a nutritionist is warranted any time a child has an atypical dietary pattern. Removal of a food group or a significant number of foods can put a child at risk for a nutrient deficiency

Early studies evaluating the effect of food additives on hyperactivity were poorly controlled and therefore added nothing to our knowledge about this issue. More recent studies investigating food dyes, food flavoring, preservatives, MSG, chocolate, and caffeine indicate that 5-10 percent of preschoolers with Attention Deficit and Hyperactivity Disorder (ADHD) respond favorably to dietary manipulation. The reasons for favorable response include placebo effect, changing interactions between the child with ADHD and the family due to the intensive intervention necessary to carry out the dietary restriction, or the effect of removing a food additive. Due to the widespread inclusion of these food items in our diets, complete elimination of these substances is difficult. A nutritionist can provide the nutritional counseling necessary to successfully eliminate these items from the family's diet, in addition to evaluating the child's diet to ensure adequate intake of nutrients in the face of the imposed significant restrictions. Because dietary elimination seems to be effective with only a small group of children, it is imperative that the efficacy of the dietary intervention be evaluated. Families should continue to work with other health professionals and consider utilizing other therapies that have been proven successful in most situations including behavior management, special education, and medications.

Other dietary factors can lead to behavior and learning difficulties. Research has shown that children who are malnourished and children who skip breakfast perform less well on standardized tests. Iron deficiency has been linked to decreased performance on cognitive tests and delays in psychomotor development. For all children, regular meals providing a wide variety of foods in an enjoyable setting foster a healthy, growing child who experiences enjoyable interactions with his or her family and community.

Dr. Schulz' Response:

I know that research on the effects of sugar and additives is not conclusive. I also know what the environment of classrooms is the day after Halloween, from the viewpoint of a teacher and a parent. The kids are climbing the wall! If you suspect that sugar has an adverse effect on your child, there is no harm in eliminating it and conducting your own experiment. You know too much sugar is not good for children anyway, so give it a try and chart your results. If it helps, great. If not, what have you lost?

CASE STUDY

Meg A., three years, nine months of age, has moderate motor delays resulting from a cerebral hemorrhage at birth. During infancy, she experienced recurrent upper respiratory infections and pneumonia. She frequently coughed and choked during breast and bottle feeding and did not gain weight well. Her mother was quite concerned that Meg did not enjoy mealtime due to frequent crying and fussing both during and after a feeding. There was also a concern that Meg was aspirating some of the fluid that she was drinking.

At approximately three years of age, Meg was evaluated by an interdisciplinary feeding team and the decision was made to place a gastrostomy tube. Since placement of the tube, Meg has been quite healthy and is currently growing along the 25-50th percentile in both height and weight. She has continued to receive oral motor stimulation that involves tastes of preferred foods and the use of the pacifier to maintain her ability to suck and swallow. Her mother often stimulates her sense of smell, taste, sight, and movement by providing firm touch around and in her mouth while naming her facial features. Meg enjoys these activities. She particularly enjoys small tastes of food and thickened liquids. Because of these small successes, Mrs. A. has expressed an interest in beginning the transition from tube to oral feeds. She has also requested that the school begin offering her small bits of food at snack and lunch time. This allows Meg more opportunities for practice and the chance to share in the social interactions that occur at lunch time. She would like Meg to sit at the table with the other youngsters in the classroom and participate in the mealtime activity to the greatest extent possible.

Prior to this request, the school personnel had been including Meg in snack and lunch by allowing her to help prepare and serve the foods and sit at the table. She receives all her nutrition during the school day through her tube. Their concerns about offering food and drink involve the safety of presenting foods to a youngster who has had such limited exposure to oral feeding. They are concerned for Meg's safety and health and there are questions of liability if Meg aspirates or becomes ill as a result of the feeding situation. They are also concerned about the time it may take to develop and implement a comprehensive feeding program and their ability to monitor her progress in the program.

Following the Individual Education Plan (IEP) meeting with Meg's school team, Mrs. A. requested a feeding clinic appointment to address the concerns of the school team. During the evaluation, there were no clinical signs of aspiration; however, Mrs. A. requested that a test (videofluoroscopy) be scheduled to further rule out the aspiration. The videofluoroscopy demonstrated that Meg was at risk to aspirate thin liquids and that as the study progressed fatigue became a contributing factor. Her position, as well as the timing of the bites, significantly affected her ability to swallow safely.

As a result of the study and at the request of the school personnel, the feeding team conducted the follow-up appointment at the school. The following issues were discussed: safety of feeding at school, positioning during feeding to minimize the likelihood of aspiration, quantity and types of foods to be offered, timing of bites, and the training needs of school personnel. A protocol was developed with input from the entire team. Mrs. A. contributed information about the size of bite, how to present the bite, and a list of Meg's favorite foods and textures. The nurse on the feeding team developed a checklist for maximizing safety during feeding that addressed what to do if she choked. The occupational therapist outlined positioning and oral motor techniques to maximize Meg's ability to chew and swallow.

The school and feeding team established an overall goal to increase the number of bites, expand the types of foods offered, and increase the texture tolerated. The first step was to offer three to five bites of preferred foods at school during snack and mealtime. Starting slowly with preferred foods allowed school personnel to work on bite size and timing of presentation with Meg's favorite foods, while not tiring Meg. This strategy was designed to create the most positive experience for the school personnel and Meg, while the school team gained experience and confidence feeding Meg.

The professionals and paraprofessionals involved with feeding Meg were also trained in positioning and feeding techniques that seemed to work best for Meg. Evaluation was a key component of the plan and the data collected (i.e., amount of food consumed, types of foods offered, and frequency of coughing and choking) assisted the team in determining when to increase the number of bites or texture of foods offered. Meg's progress would be shared among community and diagnostic team members via e-mail and videotapes and a follow-up appointment was scheduled in one month.

There are a number of instances in this scenario where communication could have broken down resulting in a very different outcome. These excellent results are the consequence of the team listening and responding to the concerns of all its members. An experienced team can predict where breakdown among diverse parties could occur and take steps to prevent this. For example, scheduling the follow-up appointment at the school helped ensure recommendations were realistic to that classroom setting. Consideration of alternative goals and compromise can lead to positive outcomes. Even though Mrs. A. wanted Meg to be fed a full snack and lunch at school, she was willing to start with three to five bites of food and move toward full meals. She listened to the concerns of the school personnel, requested a meeting with them and the hospital based feeding team, and considered alternative methods for achieving her goals based on the input of other team members.

At the one month follow-up appointment, Meg was being fed almost the entire snack and half the lunch offered to the other youngsters. Steady progress was being made in increasing both the texture and volume of foods offered. To compensate for this increase in oral feeds, the nutritionist reduced the quantity of her tube feedings and offered suggestions on the types of foods that would best meet Meg's nutritional needs. Weighing twice a month was added to the outcome measures in order to monitor the effects of the reduction in tube feedings and concomitant increase in oral feedings.

Editor's Note:

McCamman and Rues address many important issues in this chapter. One point deserving additional attention is the use of food as reinforcers. In the past, professionals have frequently recommended edibles as reinforcement for desired behaviors. This practice must be questioned given its potentially negative effects on food intake, weight gain ... We suggest that parents and professionals alike consider the value of social and other non-edible reinforcers. If foods are chosen to reinforce behaviors, those with nutritional value are preferred and a systematic plan to shift to nonedibles should be developed.

REFERENCES

Ault, M. M., Guy, B., Rues, J., Noto, L., & Guess, D. (1994). Some educational implications for students with profound disabilities at risk for inadequate nutrition and the nontherapeutic effects of medication. *Mental Retardation, 32*, 200-205.

Ault, M. M., Guy, B., & Rues, J. (1992). Nutrition analysis. In B. Guy, M. M. Ault, and D. Guess, *Analyzing behavior state in learning environments: Project ABLE*. Lawrence, KS: University of Kansas, Department of Special Education.

Horsley, J. W. (1988) Nutrition services for children with special health care needs within the public school system. *Topics in Clinical Nutrition, 3*, 55-60.

McCamman, S., & Rues, J. (1990). Nutrition monitoring and supplementation. In J. C. Graff, M. M. Ault, D. Guess, M. Taylor, & B. Thompson, *Health care for students with disabilities: An illustrated medical guide for the classroom* (pp. 79-117). Baltimore: Paul H. Brookes.

Nickel, R. E. (1996). Controversial therapies for young children with developmental disabilities. *Infants and Young Children, 8*, 29-40.

Palmer, S. (1978). Nutrition and developmental disorders: An overview. In S. Palmer & S. Ekvall (Eds.), *Pediatric nutrition in developmental disorders*, (pp. 21-24), Springfield, IL: Charles C Thomas.

Peakes, S., & Lamb, M. W. (1951). Comments on the dietary practice of cerebral palsied children. *Journal of the American Dietetic Association, 27*, 870-876.

Pfeiffer, S. I., Norton, J., Nelson, L., & Shott, S. (1995). Efficacy of vitamin B and magnesium in the treatment of autism: A methodological review and summary of outcomes. *Journal of Autism and Developmental Disorders, 25*, 481-493.

Turnbull, A. P., & Turnbull, H. R., III (1997). *Families, professionals, and exceptionality: A special partnership* (3rd ed.). New Jersey: Prentice Hall, Simon and Schuster.

Chapter 5

NURSING

Carolyn Graff

MAJOR ROLES AND RESPONSIBILITIES PLAYED BY NURSING

Nursing Practice

Nursing is a helping profession that contributes to the health and well-being of others (American Nurses Association, 1965). Nurses provide comfort and support, listen, evaluate, and intervene when necessary. They promote health by assisting children and their families to understand and cope with health problems. Nurses know when and how to use resources to help children and families move toward recovery. They coordinate various services that affect the health of others, and supervise, teach, and direct others involved in providing nursing care (*American Journal of Nursing*, 1965).

Nurses practice in a variety of settings and have many different roles and responsibilities in those settings. Nurse practice acts are established in each state and provide specific legal regulations for the practice of nursing. Each nurse practice act regulates licensure by defining the scope of nursing practice in that state.

Standards of Practice

The American Nurses Association (ANA) has established standards of practice which serve as guidelines for nurses. Based on these standards, children and their families can be assured that they are receiving high-quality care, that nurses know what is necessary to give nursing care, and that administrators can determine that care meets acceptable standards. ANA standards (Table 5-1) of clinical practice apply to the practice of all professional nurses.

62

Table 5-1
STANDARDS OF CLINICAL NURSING PRACTICE

Standards of Professional Performance
- The nurse systematically evaluates the quality and effectiveness of nursing practice.
- The nurse evaluates his/her own nursing practice in relation to professional practice standards and relevant statutes and regulations.
- The nurse acquires and maintains current knowledge in nursing practice.
- The nurse contributes to the professional development of peers, colleagues, and others.
- The nurse's decisions and actions on behalf of clients are determined in an ethical manner.
- The nurse collaborates with the client, significant others, and health care providers in providing client care.
- The nurse uses research findings in practice.
- The nurse considers factors related to safety, effectiveness, and cost in planning and delivering client care.

Note. From American Nurses Association. (1991). Standards of clinical nursing practice. Kansas City, MO: American Nurses Association.

Standards have been developed for nurses working with infants and young children under three years of age who have special health care needs (California Nurses Association, 1990; National Standards of Nursing Practice for Early Intervention Services, 1991). These standards delineate the nurse's role and responsibilities as a member of a team of professionals working with young children and their families. Their purpose was to "fulfill the profession's obligation to assure a means of improving quality care" (National Standards of Nursing Practice for Early Intervention Services, 1991).

The Nursing Process

Nurses provide expertise to teams of professionals working with children with disabilities through a method of problem identification and problem-solving. The steps of the nursing process are assessment, diagnosis (problem identification), planning (with outcome development), implementation, and evaluation.

Assessment

Nurses collect data through interview and health history, physical assessment, developmental assessment, observations of social interactions, and laboratory data. Nurses interview the child, parents, and other significant individuals to obtain a history of the child's health. Special considerations are given to the child's developmental level during an interview with a child. The health history usually follows a format as described in Table 5-2.

Table 5-2
HISTORY TAKING OUTLINE

Pediatric History Outline
Demographic Data
Reason for Seeking Health Care (Chief Complaint)
Present Illness
Family Profile
Past Health History
Immunizations
Developmental History
Review of Systems

From: Hadley, J. S. (1994). Assessing child health. In C. L. Betz, M. M. Hunsberger, & S. Wright (Eds.), *Family-centered nursing care of children* (2nd ed.) (pp. 458-512).

Physical assessment includes obtaining height, weight, head circumference, vital signs (temperature, pulse, respiration, blood pressure), and a physical examination. Developmental screening is carried out in an attempt to identify children who may need further diagnostic assessment. Nurses may assess development to determine the presence of a delay or disability, identify strengths and needs of the child and family, and suggest strategies for intervention.

Assessment of a child's nutritional status includes obtaining historical data (diet history, medical history, socioeconomic history, medication history), a clinical evaluation (physical examination), and laboratory testing to detect anemia or evaluate protein status. Although the nurse has knowledge and skills for intervention with some nutritional problems, the registered dietitian/nutritionist has extensive training in nutrition and is consulted when the problem is beyond the level of the nurse's abilities (Ott, 1994) (see Chapter 4).

Laboratory screening tests that may be recommended by the nurse include hematocrit, hemoglobin, Sickledex, phenylketonuria (PKU) testing, and lead screening. Hemoglobin and hematocrit are done when there is a concern about anemia based on the history or physical examination. Sickledex is a screening test for sickle cell anemia, and PKU testing is mandatory testing on all newborns in most states. Screening for lead toxicity can be done by testing blood and urine (Wonnacott, 1994).

Nursing Diagnosis

Nursing diagnosis is the identification of the child's or family's problem or concern. It is the nurse's clinical judgment about the responses of the child or family to actual or potential health problems or life processes. Nursing diagnosis provides the basis for selecting nursing interventions to reach outcomes for which the nurse is accountable (North American Nursing Diagnosis Association, 1994).

Nursing practice is dependent, interdependent, and independent. Dependent activities are those areas that the nurse is accountable for based on the regimen prescribed by the physician. Interdependent activities are those areas of nursing practice in which the responsibility and accountability of the nurse, physician, or other disciplines overlap and require collaboration between two or more disciplines. Independent activities are those areas that are the direct responsibility of the nurse. Nursing diagnoses reflect the interdependent and independent dimensions of nursing (Wong, 1997).

Collaborative problems (Carpenito, 1995) are problems of the child or family that usually require a collaborative approach to prevention, treatment, or intervention. Disciplines such as audiology, medicine, nutrition, occupational therapy, physical therapy, psychology, respiratory therapy, and speech language pathology may be consulted by the nurse to provide the necessary services (screening, assessment, intervention, or treatment) (Wong, 1997).

Planning

In the planning step, the nurse identifies the goals or outcomes with the child, parents, family, or a combination of these. The goal or outcome is the desired change in the child's condition or behavior that is agreed on by the child or family (or both) and nurse. Goals are developed according to the strengths and needs of the child and family (Wong, 1997).

Implementation

This refers to the nursing interventions or actions the nurse takes based on the nurse's knowledge and reasoning process. It is the actual delivery of nursing care to the child or family. Nurse's activities are guided by the child's current status and nursing and medical diagnoses.

Evaluation

In the last step, evaluation may be an ongoing part of the intervention. The nurse asks, "Did the intervention work?" "Is the child making progress toward the outcome?" "If not, why?" Evaluation is most effective when the child's and family's input is obtained and used to make modifications in the plan. The nurse working with young children may have difficulty evaluating the intervention because of the age of the child and the child's limitations in cognitive development. The nurse then finds it necessary to validate perceptions with the child's parents and family (Betz et al., 1994).

The nursing process is a continuous cycle. The nurse uses each interaction with the child and family to continue assessing and reassessing the nursing diagnoses and plan. Written documentation of nurses' interventions and the child's response is required.

CONTRIBUTIONS OF NURSING TO
INTERDISCIPLINARY PRACTICE

While standards of practice guide nurses, settings of practice influence nurses' roles and responsibilities. Nurses working with children with disabilities may work in hospitals, homes, schools, or clinics. These nurses' roles may include case finding, direct care-giving, teaching, providing guidance and support, consulting, coordinating, collaborating with other professionals, and being a child and family advocate (Betz et al, 1993).

Case Finding

The term *case finding* has been used in public health practice to refer to the process of identifying persons who need assistance or information. Although this has usually referred to nurses working in the community, nurses working in the hospital may also be involved in this activity. Because diseases can be prevented or minimized with early identification and treatment, case finding and early identification have been major responsibilities for nurses according to Barnard and Erickson (as cited in Russell & Free, 1994) and Krajicek and Tomlinson (as cited in Russell & Free, 1994). Nurses are often the first health care professionals to have contact with children and families and are in excellent positions to identify problems or potential problems of children and families. For example, nurses in hospital full term nurseries or neonatal intensive care units (NICUs) may recognize minor abnormalities that can be brought to the attention of other professionals for further evaluation.

Methods used to identify children at risk or children who have developmental difficulties include screenings of health and development. Screenings are carried out to identify a potential problem and to indicate a child's strengths and needs. Screenings are not done to make a diagnosis.

Health screening may be conducted in the school, clinic, or home. General health screenings are carried out by a nurse practitioner, clinical nursing specialist, or physician on a regular basis. Nurses may be responsible for carrying out the general health screening along with auditory, visual, and general developmental screening.

In addition to their responsibility to recognize children who are at risk for developmental and health problems, nurses have responsibilities to identify any problems associated with a disability or problems that are present in addition to the disability. Nurses should not only identify problems associated with a disability but identify ways to prevent and reduce associated problems. All behaviors and needs of children with disabilities are not related to the disability. Children with disabilities have typical childhood illnesses. In other words, nurses must look and think beyond the child's disability.

Direct Care Giving

Nurses working in hospitals should adapt their care to fit the specific needs of the child. The plan of care should allow for (a) recognition of the child's expressed needs and concerns (at whatever developmental level), (b) support for the child's move to a higher level of independence (as possible), and (c) progress at the child's own rate.

During hospitalization, the nurse may be the person who feeds the child and assists the child with dressing and toileting. The nurse communicates often with the child during various care-giving activities (e.g., feeding, administering medications, or dressing changes). Also, the nurse communicates closely with other professionals to assure that the technique used during feeding is appropriate, that the position for feeding is appropriate, and that the nurse's level of communication is appropriate for the child's level of communication.

The nurse will be involved with position changes during the hospitalization to avoid prolonged pressure on various parts of the child's body. This will likely be done every two hours along with careful checks of the skin for signs of redness and application of preventive measures as needed. Equipment such as special mattresses may be needed during the hospitalization or special equipment may be used on wheelchairs to equalize pressure.

Close work with the occupational therapist, physical therapist, pediatric physiatrist, and family will lead to successful problem-solving in this area.

An understanding of the child's elimination patterns and habits is necessary to prevent alteration of the usual pattern during hospitalization. If a routine, healthy pattern has not been established, this can be addressed during the hospitalization. Working with the nutritionist, the nurse and family can determine whether dietary adjustments can be made to manage constipation and diarrhea. Additionally, inadequate fluid intake may be an issue for some children. Creative strategies may be tried during the hospitalization to best encourage a child's safe fluid intake.

Home health nurses provide nursing care to children discharged from a hospital or to children requiring a level of care that can be given safely in the home. Home health care may be provided through hospitals, visiting nurse associations, public health nursing agencies, hospices, and private home care agencies.

Nurses work to promote optimal activities of daily living as developmentally appropriate. Following hospitalization for surgery, the child's level of participation with dressing, eating, or toileting may be diminished. Physical therapists can assist with increasing mobility and occupational therapists can assist with promoting activities of daily living. Nurses should be aware of the activities that the child can safely do and create opportunities in the hospital and home for the child to participate in these activities. It is important that the family be supported in their efforts to promote the child's independence which, in turn, promotes the child's self-esteem.

Teaching

As teachers, nurses explain concepts and facts about health, demonstrate procedures of care, determine that the child and family understand, reinforce learning, and evaluate progress in learning. Nurses structure health teaching to incorporate the family's values and health beliefs. They use teaching methods that match the child's or family's abilities and needs and incorporate other resources such as extended family, friends, and neighbors, as desired by the child and parents. Nurses may teach the child how to perform care alone or teach the parent, school staff, or others to provide needed care. This may involve demonstrating how to carry out a specific type of care. Nurses may encourage parents to allow their child to carry out certain aspects of self care to promote self-esteem and increase long-term likelihood that the child will continue to provide the necessary care.

Procedures such as surgery or diagnostic tests should be explained to the child in terms the child can understand. Working with the child's parents, nurses can determine what method and level of explanation will be most effective for the child.

Nurses work to prevent illnesses to which children may be vulnerable. They provide education on the transmission of communicable diseases and how to prevent illnesses through immunizations, good hand washing, skin care, and avoiding infectious contacts. They encourage early and adequate prenatal care and a healthy lifestyle during pregnancy (e.g., avoiding use of alcohol during pregnancy) (Russell & Free, 1994).

Nurses provide families with information about their child's condition, with the understanding that the family is the expert on the child's personality and environment and on the context of the child's family life (Clarke, 1994). Nurses must continue to expand their knowledge of childhood disabilities and risk factors for children and families.

Providing Guidance and Support

Nurses are in excellent positions to offer support to the child with a disability and the family. They may be available in the hospital when family members receive a new diagnosis and can make referrals to others in the hospital or community. Nurses should be aware of community resources for families, supports such as parent groups, information networks, and groups or agencies where services are centralized. Additionally, nurses are responsible for helping parents access resources in the community. Resources such as Supplemental Security Income (SSI) can offer financial support to families.

Nurses can help families find highly skilled health care professionals who enjoy providing health care to children with disabilities. The nurse may facilitate visits to another health care professional by sharing information about the child with the parents' approval. This information may include the child's ability to communicate, the child's physical disabilities and use of a wheelchair or other equipment, financial arrangements and problem behaviors, along with tips to deal with these behaviors.

Interpreting medical information and professional jargon to families and other professionals is often a nursing responsibility. Nurses should have a clear understanding of what is being shared and inform the family if there is not a clear understanding of this information. Careful listening and observing are very important when parents ask questions. Parents may have questions produced by feelings of hurt, despair, or anger. It is important to answer questions factually and with great concern and care.

Nurses must examine their own feelings of fear, discomfort, anger, or inadequacy when working with children with disabilities. The child and family will sense emotions and attitudes behind the nurse's actions. The nurse must "see the person" by looking beyond the disability and sensitively acknowledge their own feelings.

Nurses may be extremely helpful in assisting with identifying ways to fit a health care procedure into the life of a child and family. The goal is to minimize the impact of the procedure on the child's and family's routines and lifestyle.

Nurses provide comfort by demonstrating care to the child and family as individuals with unique feelings and needs. Nurses help the child and family reach their own goals rather than encouraging emotional or physical dependence (Perry, 1997).

Consulting

Nurses may provide health care consultation services by practicing with other nurses and other health care professionals who provide care to groups of children who are well or whose health status is stable. Nurses in schools often provide consultation to school staff about certain health-related procedures (e.g., seizure monitoring, monitoring shunts, clean intermittent catheterization, or gastrostomy tube feedings). School districts vary widely in their ability to provide school nursing services. When a nurse cannot be employed full time for a school, a health aide, parent volunteer, or school clerical staff person may be the designated provider of health care. The school nurse visits the school regularly, providing information and guidance.

Coordinating

In hospitals in which complex care is provided by numerous professionals, nurses will coordinate the activities of other members of the health team to offer smoother, less repetitive, and more time- and cost-efficient services to a child and family. Nurses may help families "navigate" through the maze that sometimes surrounds health care. *Case manager* may be the term used for a nurse working in these roles.

Collaborating with Other Professionals

Nurses working to assist families reach their goals must be committed to the family's goals and values. Nursing roles allow the family and nurse to be full and equal participants in the plan for the child's and family's care. It is important to collaborate with the family to design a flexible family plan that may be modified once the child is at home (Clarke, 1994).

Nurses frequently refer the child and family to other professionals and agencies for assistance that is beyond the scope of nursing practice. The basis of this referral hinges on the individual nurse's understanding of the knowledge, skills, and abilities of other professionals. In their effort to address the holistic health care needs of the child and family, nurses may use strategies to restore emotional, spiritual, and social well-being of the child and family. They help the child and family set goals and reach these goals with the least expense of cost and time.

Nurses are perhaps the best prepared team member to understand the relationships between health, medications, independence, and function. Nurses have much experience with health, using both medical and nonmedical approaches. Because of their education about medications, ways of facilitating health, and understanding how the child functions in the environment, nurses are often interpreters for other members of the team about the effects of medication on the child (Barks, 1994).

Advocate

As advocate, the nurse works with the family to decide about health care and to be a spokesperson for the child who is unable to make care needs known. Although the nurse may be the primary advocate for the child or for a family, most often the nurse joins with the family and other health care professionals to advocate for obtaining optimal services (Betz et al., 1994). The role of the advocate is to help the child and family remain independent and not foster or promote dependence.

When making recommendations to families about the type of care needed, nurses should consider the cost (financial, emotional, and time) to the family. It is important for nurses to clarify within themselves, with the family, and with other professionals, the real need for a given recommendation. Once a recommendation for care has been made, the nurse must support the family in following through with the recommended care. This may involve helping families access resource lists or sharing of information.

Because siblings are an important part of the child's development, nurses must consider siblings of the child with a disability. The child with special needs should be included in the siblings' circle of friends. Siblings may need explanations about the care a child receives and may appreciate the opportunity to participate, to some extent, with this care. They may need preparation for teasing of their sibling with a disability and strategies to handle those situations. Strategies and activities for siblings have been described by Meyer and Vadasy (1994). These include sibshops which offer opportunities for siblings to meet other siblings of children with special needs and share their perspectives and experiences.

THE ROLES PARENTS TYPICALLY PLAY IN THE OPTIMAL INTERDISCIPLINARY SERVICE PROVISION OF NURSING

Nurses view the family as the recipient of nursing care. The family is seen as the essential environment for the child. While the focus of nursing care is usually on the child, consideration is given to family needs, goals, and priorities. The child cannot be understood unless viewed within the context of the entire family (Clarke, 1994).

According to Harkins (1994), the goals of nurses working with a child with a chronic illness and the family include: (1) assisting the child and family in the psychosocial adaptation to the child's illness, (2) promoting optimal potential for the child's and family's growth and development, and (3) encouraging families to make appropriate use of resources within the health care system.

In assisting with the psychosocial adaptation to the child's illness, the nurse must focus on caring for the developmental needs of the child and family, as well as on the illness and its effects on the family. Nurses can assist the child and family to develop realistic goals, facilitate mourning, and promote the child's self-worth. They can encourage progress along the normal developmental trajectory toward independence and develop open channels of communication among parents, child, and health care system.

Parents must be willing to share their knowledge about their child, including their child's strengths and limitations. It is important that parents share the difficulties they experience in providing care. Although nurses may vary in their ability to portray openness and willingness to listen and learn from the parent, parents must respect their own views and observations and knowledge of their child and share these with others. When parents share this information with nurses, it can be helpful to be aware that nurses may be dealing with some of their own feelings about working with the child. These feelings may include fear, discomfort, or anger.

Nurses are individuals with their own values and perspectives. They may expect open, revealing conversations with parents about their children because their own families communicated in this way. Or, they may be surprised when parents are open and revealing in their conversations because their own families did not communicate in this way. If parents feel uncomfortable in communicating with a nurse, it is important to share this discomfort with the nurse.

The nurse's goal is to establish an atmosphere that encourages communication and leads to independent family functioning and problem-solving. A nurse's restating or reflecting on something the parent has said is often their effort to clarify the issues further or facilitate decision-making by parents. It may be helpful for parents to restate their view in an attempt to inform the nurse what their perspective is. If decisions have been made that parents are uncertain about, they should inform the nurse directly about this uncertainty.

Nurses may need to be reminded that parents do not always agree with each other about decisions related to their child's care. Nurses should respect each parent's point of view and encourage expression of these views. The nurse's goal is empowerment of the family with decreasing dependence on the health care provider and with families increasing responsibility for their own health care. If the nurse's perceptions are incorrect, parents should tell the nurse immediately. For example, if the family is ready to take some responsibility for care of a child, but still needs help or feels uncertain about aspects of a child's care, it is important to speak out and inform the nurse. On the other hand, with efforts to share all aspects of a particular procedure or type of care with parents, the nurse may overlook many aspects that the parent already knows. If this is the case and parents feel as if the nurse is not recognizing how much they already know, parents should talk directly with the nurse.

During the history-taking process, if parents are asked questions they do not understand, they must tell the nurse. Parents can restate the question and ask, "Is this . . . what you mean?" If a question is offensive, it is important for parents to speak up and inform the nurse that they feel uncomfortable with the question.

A nurse may make assumptions about a child's or family's ethnicity based on the nurse's reading about characteristics of an ethnic group in a textbook or based on the nurse's own past experiences. These assumptions may be factual or distorted. Parents' careful explanations of a particular health care belief or reasons for a unique method of treatment can inform the nurse of the family's own approaches to the child's care. Differences between the nurse and parents can lead to opportunities for greater understanding and growth. The nurse and parents may recognize the unique aspects of the family and the richness of one's own and another's ethnicity by sharing these ideas.

Nurses may expect the parents to be available during a child's hospitalization to provide a stable and supportive environment for the child, to interpret the child's behavior to others, and to assist with communicating with the child. Parents also need to be available to learn care that will be given at home, to provide consent for treatment to the child, and to actually assist with care of the child. It will be important for parents to share as much information as they feel comfortable with about why a family member may not be able to stay with the child. Nurses care for and about children and want to know that their parents do, too. Nurses feel responsible and have responsibilities to share information about a child's care with the parents and usual caregivers. The nurse's sharing of information is not intended to take the role of the parent or to indicate that the nurse always knows what is best for the child.

TYPICAL PARENT QUESTIONS/COMMENTS FOR NURSING

Why do professionals try to paint a positive picture when parents need to know the bottom line?

Nurses may have difficulty sharing information in a direct manner with parents for numerous reasons. For one, they may have difficulty because they imagine how they, themselves, would feel if they were in the parents' position. They may find the thought of being in the parents' position overwhelming. Parents often do feel overwhelmed with what is going on for them and their child and family. When an overwhelmed nurse meets an overwhelmed family, each may talk around the facts. The nurse has the information that needs to be delivered to the family. In that respect, the nurse has a sense of control. In an effort to be kind to the family, the nurse may choose to be easy with the family and not give all the information at once. The nurse may present some of the facts or only positive facts in the beginning. The nurse may be apologetic that the information has to be shared at all.

Painting a positive picture, when both positive and negative aspects need to be shared, is likely related to the professional's view that parents will have difficulty with the information. The nurse's hesitation in sharing has an air of presumption that the family will not want to hear what is said or may not be able or ready to handle the information. Families may already know or sense what is going to be said by the nurse. The parent or family member may have a partial or unclear view or perception of the picture. Open communication and sharing can lead to a clearer picture of the issues being faced by the child and family.

I've been frustrated with the medical community's inability to provide current information about relatively common disorders (e.g., Down syndrome). How do medical personnel keep themselves current and what can be done to assure that this happens?

Renewal of a nurse's license to practice in some states depends on the nurse obtaining continuing education. An issue may be the limited opportunities for nurses to gain new knowledge and information about childhood disabilities.

In a publication edited by Austin and Donohoe (1996), the continuing education needs of nurses who provide care for children with special health care needs was addressed. Although the knowledge base of nursing education is vast, it must include pediatric content that focuses on the child's and family's needs and available resources in the community. The ability to access and disseminate information is vital to coping with the health care knowledge explosion and can lead to networking of nurses in the community.

Continuing education is viewed as a professional responsibility. "Each nurse is responsible to develop service skills and achieve mastery of telecommunication technologies. The challenge to identify and utilize effective, comprehensive systems, access resources, solutions, and interdisciplinary supports remains a professional responsibility of each nurse" (Austin & Donohoe, 1996, p. 31). Federal support was considered vital to developing computer-assisted technology for continuing education. As the professional nurse cares for children with special health care needs, and negotiates the managed care and evolving health care systems, the demand for continuing education continues to be a priority to assure quality care (Austin & Donohoe, 1996).

I'm frustrated with school personnel's reluctance to perform simple procedures for my child without the presence of a nurse (e.g., administration of medications). What kind of medically related things would you consider "out-of-bounds" for school personnel?

School personnel's ability to perform procedures are established by policies for each school district. More importantly, school nurses perform procedures as allowed by each state's nurse practice act. Nurses may delegate some nursing procedures to nonnursing personnel depending on the provisions in the state's nurse practice act.

Statements regarding delegation of nursing responsibilities to nonnursing school personnel have been published by the National Association of State School Nurse Consultants (1995). As noted in this document, "Nursing activities are defined by state statute and interpreted by the state board of nursing. A state's attorney general's opinion, court decision or other mandate may modify the state's definition of nursing or interpretation of its scope of practice. On the basis of these definitions and interpretations, the nurse decides whether the activity or procedure is one that can be performed only by a registered nurse (RN)" (National Association of State School Nurse Consultants, 1995). Delegation of nursing activities may be appropriate when it is not prohibited by state statute or regulations, legal interpretations, or agency policies. It does not require exercising nursing judgment and it is delegated and supervised by an RN.

School nurses develop an individualized health care plan (IHCP) for the student with special health care needs. The assessment includes a brief health history, identification of special health care needs, baseline health status, medication, diet/nutrition, transportation, equipment, and possible problems and interventions. Planning includes establishing emergency plans for school and transportation; notifying the fire department, emergency medical transport system, and local emergency room of possible student emergency needs; review of the IHCP by physician, signature by parent, educational administrator, and school nurse; and incorporation of the IHCP into student records as appropriate (Palfrey, Haynie, Porter, Bierle, Cooperman, & Lowcock, 1992).

Administration of medications is a common activity or procedure that occurs in schools. Nurses must refer to their state practice acts to determine who administers medications in schools and what medications are restricted. Recommendations in this area have been issued by the National Association of School Nurses, Inc. (Schwab, 1991), National Association of State School Nurse Consultants (1995), and Porter, Haynie, Bierle, Caldwell, and Palfrey (1997).

Porter et al. (1997) suggest that the IHCP should include certain information about the student who is to receive medication at school. The IHCP should: (a) designate the individual responsible for dispensing medication, (b) list medications administered at home, (c) list medications needed at school, (d) indicate dose and time of medication administration, (e) list medication side effects and interaction effects that may affect school functioning or child's safety, (f) list any adverse reactions to the medication the child may have experienced and appropriate responses, (g) identify medications that are administered on an as-needed basis and the circumstances that indicate the medication is needed, (h) indicate known allergies, and (i) delineate protocols for administering experimental medications (Porter et al., 1997).

CASE EXAMPLE

Karen walks into Bruce S.'s room to adjust the intravenous (IV) fluids and check his vital signs. It is now two days since the diagnosis of cerebral palsy (CP) has been discussed with Bruce's parents. They appeared numb after this news had been shared with them. Mr. S. sat at the foot of Bruce's crib and occasionally had moist eyes. Bruce is Mr. and Mrs. S.'s second child. He is five months old. Mrs. S. has taken a very matter-of-fact approach to her son's new diagnosis and takes notes on a small pad. She is a reporter for a local newspaper.

Karen, the nurse, adjusts Bruce's IV and turns to Mr. and Mrs. S. Mrs. S. smiles and talks about Bruce's vital signs and his respiratory status. His breath sounds are still coarse, but his temperature and oxygen saturation level are normal. Karen and Mrs. S. discuss results of the latest chest x-ray and evidence that Bruce's pneumonia is clearing.

Bruce has been hospitalized for three days with pneumonia. His ten-year-old sister, Ashley, was helping feed him when he choked. According to the chest x-ray, Bruce aspirated formula. He has been hospitalized to clear up the pneumonia and consider whether feedings by bottle are appropriate for him. He has received antibiotics along with medication and treatments to assist with breathing. Today his physician has presented the news that a gastrostomy tube is a possibility. Mrs. S. is ready to have a tube placed.

Mr. S. wants his son to eat and does not want a tube extending out of Bruce's stomach. Mr. and Mrs. S. are busy trying to keep things going at their jobs and assure that Ashley's life continues in a somewhat normal fashion. They have had no time to talk about the possibility of a gastrostomy tube and the diagnosis of cerebral palsy.

Karen and Mrs. S. begin an upbeat conversation about how well Bruce is doing today compared to yesterday. They comment on all aspects of his care and Mrs. S. indicates that she is ready to go ahead with the surgery to place a gastrostomy tube. Mr. S. does not speak. Karen, the nurse, laughs as she leaves and does not acknowledge the pained look on Mr. S.'s face.

After Karen left, Mrs. S. comments on Mr. S.'s silence. He erupts, "You make all the decisions here! I am tired of this! It is as if what I think and say makes no difference." Mrs. S. becomes quiet and looks at her husband with sad, tearful eyes. "I do not want to take over. I am so tired of this. First, finding out that Bruce has cerebral palsy. Now, we have to make a decision about surgery. We have no choice but to go ahead with it."

"Sure we have choices," Mr. S. said. "We can continue to feed him very carefully and find new ways to feed him. The feeding specialists are coming this afternoon. They will figure out a way to feed him so we do not have to put him through that surgery."

"Who is going to be feeding him? Do you expect me to quit my job?" replied Mrs. S. "We cannot manage without my salary and my health insurance!"

"Of course not. We will take turns and make it work. I can change my hours to work at home during the morning and early afternoon until you get home. Then you can take over," Mr. S. proposes.

Mrs. S. asks, "When will we spend time with Ashley? She needs our time and attention right now."

"Well, we can only do so much. I will ask my mother to help us too. She won't mind," Mr. S. offers. Mrs. S. looks down toward the floor. They sit quietly while Bruce sleeps.

Marianne enters the room. She is the nurse who works in the evening and has been wonderful according to Mr. S. She greets Mr. and Mrs. S. and asks how long Bruce has been sleeping. Marianne asks Mr. and Mrs. S. how each of them is today. They both look tired and begin talking. Mr. S. explains his hesitation about the gastrostomy tube and the differences between his point of view and Mrs. S.'s point of view. They ask Marianne what Bruce will really be like when he is older, two years, three years, or four years. Marianne answers honestly that she does not know. She does know that Bruce's brain tissue has been damaged. The cause of this damage is not known. All evaluations and tests that have been done give no clues to what caused this damage. More laboratory tests may be recommended to look for a cause.

Marianne then checks Bruce's vital signs, IV fluid rate, IV site, skin color, and breathing. She then sits down and begins to share what she has just found from her assessment. Bruce is looking better than the day before. His breathing is more relaxed, easier, and less rapid. His oxygen saturation rate is within normal limits.

Marianne leaves Bruce's room and calls Bruce's physician. She clarifies the question of what is going on with Bruce with his physician. Marianne describes Bruce's improvements based on her assessment and indicates that she will discuss a parent networking group with Mr. and Mrs. S. She reports that the couple has differences in their ideas about the gastrostomy tube. In fact, Mr. S. wants to view a videotape about gastrostomy tubes and making the decision for placement of these tubes.

Later, the physician visits and discusses each option (surgical placement of a gastrostomy tube or feeding with no tube placement). Marianne also discusses the resources of home health nursing and early intervention services that are available for Bruce. Mrs. S. says that Bruce has been involved with a parent education program as his older sister was in her early years of life. These parent educators have visited Bruce twice and had questioned whether Bruce's development was delayed. These educators contacted the early intervention program and a teacher had made one visit to the S. home. Mrs. S. says the early intervention staff will continue to visit Bruce after his discharge from the hospital.

Bruce has the gastrostomy tube placed and does well following surgery. Both Mr. and Mrs. S. have learned to take care of Bruce's gastrostomy tube. They know how to administer the tube feeding, what to do to take care of Bruce's skin around the tube, signs of problems that may occur, and what to do about these problems.

Ashley has not helped with her brother's care. Since his return home, she watches quietly. A home health nurse, Lynn, visits Bruce and his family every day for the first few weeks after he left the hospital. She notices that Ashley is very quiet and has a sad look on her face as she watches her parents and the nurse care for and attend to Bruce.

After a few visits, in the home, Lynn begins talking with Mrs. S. about Ashley and her involvement with Bruce's care. Lynn learns of Ashley's involvement with Bruce prior to his hospitalization. She explores with Mrs.

S. the possibility of Ashley assisting with feeding Bruce by holding the formula can until it is ready to be poured into the container. Gradually, Ashley helps Lynn and her mother with Bruce's feedings. She begins talking to him again and holds his rattle so he can see and hear it as she had before his illness. Ashley does not like the tube coming out of Bruce's stomach and does not want to hold or touch him. Mrs. S. and Lynn support Ashley's position. However, Lynn talks with Ashley about what the tube means and how it works. Ashley listens carefully. A few days later, Ashley comes to Lynn and asks more questions about the tube and its purpose for Bruce. She wonders if she will ever have to have a tube like this. She asks if she made this happen to Bruce by feeding him his formula. Lynn explains that Ashley will not have to have a tube like Bruce has. Lynn speaks in a matter-of-fact manner with Ashley and carefully uses language that a ten-year-old can understand. Mrs. S. listens as Lynn talks with Ashley. She is pleased that Ashley is sharing her feelings and thoughts.

Mr. and Mrs. S. meet with other parents of children who have special needs. They go to a support group of parents involved with the early intervention program. They meet another family who has a child with a gastrostomy tube and two families who have children with cerebral palsy. During a support group meeting, Mr. and Mrs. B. tell Mr. and Mrs. S. about their difficulties with a home health nurse. The nurse told them that their child would always have a gastrostomy tube and would never be able to eat again by mouth. They went on to say that the nurse was not accurate and that their son eventually began taking food by mouth as he became healthier. Why do nurses not understand the kind of care a child needs before they talk with the family? In fact, several professionals had told the family this. How could they all be wrong?

The Bs. told Mr. and Mrs. S. that they later found out that the nurse really was uncomfortable working with their son. Their son was the first child with developmental disabilities and a gastrostomy tube with whom this nurse had worked. In the nurse's attempt to deal with her own discomfort, she used technical information and kept the conversation and discussions on a very technical level. Also, Mrs. B. said the nurse did not ask them to tell her about their child. She had the notion that she was the expert and that this family was in need of her advice. Mrs. B. said the truth was that they were, indeed, the experts on their child and wanted to tell the nurse what they knew. Mr. B. said the nurse did not ask and did not listen when he or Mrs. B. tried to tell the nurse about their child. Finally Mr. and Mrs. B. said to the nurse, "You are not comfortable with our son." Then the nurse acknowledged her level of discomfort and asked for explanations and descriptions.

Mrs. B. said, "I was really angry with this nurse. But, the truth is that the nurse was not sure about what to do. I asked myself, 'Why would she be sent here to help us when she does not understand our child's needs?' According to Mr. B., the truth was that the nurse actually knew a lot about gastrostomy tubes and the care that was needed. What she did not know was how to work with a child who had seizures, breath holding spells, and developmental delays.

Mrs. B. said, "After she told us she was not comfortable with our child, she came the next day and gave us new information about managing our son's tube feedings. She really understood what our son needed. She told us she had read and talked with the nurses who had cared for our son in the hospital to get a better understanding of what was needed. She brought us copies of articles she was reading. We all learned something about each other and the many possible ways to care for our son. It was a good experience for all of us."

Mr. and Mrs. S. found that the parent group offered a chance to share their experiences and learn from others' experiences. They seemed stronger and more prepared to deal with the issues they faced with their son and the team of professionals working with them. They also found a sense of hope and offered others the message that their fatigue would lessen over time and they would find enjoyment and satisfaction in being parents of a child with a disability.

At age three, Bruce entered a preschool program where he spent four hours a day with children who were developing typically. Therapists came to the preschool and gave the preschool staff many excellent ideas on ways to promote Bruce's development. An issue that was difficult to resolve was related to the fact that Bruce needed medication for his seizure disorder once during the school hours. The school nurse could not come to the classroom every day to give Bruce his medication. Following school district policy and the state nurse practice act, the school nurse delegated this responsibility to the paraprofessional working with Bruce. She gave him the seizure medication through the gastrostomy tube and administered the tube feeding once during the school day. The school nurse met with Mr. and Mrs. S. before Bruce began the preschool and determined how his tube feedings were carried out at home. She developed a written procedure for Bruce's tube feeding. Using this information, she taught the paraprofessional and teacher how to administer the tube feeding and went to the classroom at intervals to observe the tube feeding. She was available to come to assist in the classroom if problems arose.

Editors' Note:

Graff has done an excellent job of delineating the roles and responsibilities of nurses and families in an array of contexts. Dr. Schulz best summarizes the editorial response to the complexities of nursing raised in this chapter with the following comments:

Dr. Schulz's Comments:

When my daughter was born, the nurse who examined her noticed that she was "tongue tied" and alerted the pediatrician to the problem. It was solved immediately and prevented a possible speech difficulty in the future.

Working with siblings is such an important part of the family situation; I commend the author for addressing this issue. Another part of this issue is helping siblings deal with their friends' reactions to the child with a disability. My daughter said, "I never knew whether to explain Billy to my friends (which somehow seemed unfair to him) or to just let them form their own opinions."

In addition to education about the nature of childrens' disabilities, training should include acceptance of children with disabilities as children who are children first, rather than in terms of the disability. As one of the first persons to interact with the mother of a baby with a disability, nurses can have very positive effects on the parents or, sad to say, very negative effects.

I was asked to visit a mother who had just given birth to a baby with Down syndrome. The baby was the first born in the new year and was eligible for a number of gifts, a write-up in the local newspaper and pictures of the mother with the baby. The nurse in attendance advised the mother not to accept the award since her baby was "deformed" and she wouldn't want the picture in the paper. The mother was devastated and, in her confusion, accepted the nurse's advice.

REFERENCES

Alpern, G., Boll, T., & Shearer, M. (1986). *The developmental profile II.* Los Angeles: Western Psychological Services.

American Nurses Association. (1991). *Standards of clinical nursing practice.* Kansas City, MO: American Nurses Association.

American Nurses Association. (1965). Educational preparation for nurse practitioners. *American Journal of Nursing, 65*(12), 106.

Austin, J. R., & Donohoe, M. L. (Eds.). (1996). *Continuing education needs for nurses caring for children with special health care needs* (MCHB Grant #MCU115042). Vienna, VA: National Maternal and Child Health Clearinghouse.

Barks, L. (1994). Approaches to medication administration. In S. P. Roth & J. S. Morse (Eds.), *Life-span approach to nursing care for individuals with developmental disabilities* (pp. 193-218). Baltimore: Paul H. Brookes.

Betz, C. L., Hunsberger, M. M., & Wright, S. (1994). *Family-centered nursing care of children* (2nd ed.). Philadelphia: W. B. Saunders.

California Nurses' Association. (1990). *Nursing standards for early intervention services for children and families at risk.* San Francisco: California Nurses' Association.

Carpenito, L. J. (1995). *Nursing diagnosis application to clinical practice* (6th ed.). Philadelphia: J.B. Lippincott.

Clarke, P. N. (1994). Family theories and assessment. In C.L. Betz, M. M. Hunsberger, & S. Wright (Eds.), *Family-centered nursing care of children* (2nd ed.,) (pp. 35-67). Philadelphia: W. B. Saunders.

Hadley, J. S. (1994). Assessing child health. In C. L. Betz, M. M. Hunsberger, & S. Wright (Eds.), *Family-centered nursing care of children* (2nd ed.) (pp. 458-512). Philadelphia: W. B. Saunders.

Harkins, A. (1994). Chronic illness. In C. L. Betz, M. M. Hunsberger, & S. Wright (Eds.), *Family-centered nursing care of children* (2nd ed.) (pp. 651 -688). Philadelphia: W. B. Saunders Company.

Magyary, D., Brandt, P., Fleming, J., Kieckhefer, G., & Padgett, D. (1993). Nursing specialty practice guidelines: The implications for clinical scholarship and early intervention practice. *Journal of Pediatric Nursing, 8*(4),253-260.

Meyer, D. J., & Vadasy, P. F. (1994). *Workshops for siblings of children with special needs.* Baltimore: Paul H. Brookes.

National Association of School Nurse Consultants. (1995). Delegation of school health services to unlicensed assistive personnel: A position paper of the National Association of State School Nurse Consultants. *Journal of School Nursing, 11*(2), 17-19.

National standards of nursing practice for early intervention services. (1991). Leadership Development for Nurses in Early Intervention Project (MCJ215052). Lexington, KY: University of Kentucky, Division of Parent-Child Nursing.

North American Nursing Diagnosis Association: *Nursing diagnoses: definitions and classifications 1995-1996.* (1994). Philadelphia: NANDA.

Ott, C. B. (1994). Healthy dietary practice. In C. L. Betz, M. M. Hunsberger, & S. Wright (Eds.), *Family-centered nursing care of children* (2nd ed.) (pp. 546-600). Philadelphia: W. B. Saunders.

Palfrey, J. S., Haynie, M., Porter, S., Bierle, T., Cooperman, P., & Lowcock, J. (1992). Project school care: Integrating children assisted by medical technology into educational settings. *Journal of School Health, 62*(2), 51.

Perry, A. G. (1997). Profession of nursing. In P. A. Potter & A. G. Perry (Eds.), *Fundamentals of nursing: Concepts, process, and practice* (4th ed.) (pp. 207-231). St. Louis: C.V. Mosby.

Porter, S., Haynie, M., Bierle, T., Caldwell, T. H., Palfrey, J. S. (1997). *Children and youth assisted by medical technology in educational settings: Guidelines for care.* Baltimore: Paul H. Brookes.

Russell, F. F., & Free, T. A. (1994). Nurse's role in habilitation. In S. P. Roth & J. S. Morse (Eds.), *Life-span approach to nursing care for individuals with developmental disabilities* (pp. 59-87). Baltimore: Paul H. Brookes.

Schwab, N. (1991). *Guidelines for school nursing documentation: Standards, issues, and models.* Scarborough, Maine: National Association of School Nurses, Inc.

Wong, D. L. (1997). *Whaley & Wong's essentials of pediatric nursing* (5th ed.). St. Louis: C.V. Mosby.

Wonnacott, E. (1994). The injured child. In C. L. Betz, M. M. Hunsberger, & S. Wright (Eds.), *Family-centered nursing care of children* (2nd ed.) (pp. 2080-2126). Philadelphia: W. B. Saunders.

Chapter 6

OCCUPATIONAL THERAPY

WINNIE DUNN

The purpose of this chapter is to provide an overview of the contributions that occupational therapy can make to the interdisciplinary process when serving children with disabilities and their families. The chapter reviews the focus of occupational therapy, the contributions to interdisciplinary and family-centered care, and common concerns of parents. It also provides an example of optimal interdisciplinary services which include occupational therapy services.

MAJOR RESPONSIBILITIES AND ROLES OF OCCUPATIONAL THERAPISTS

Focus of Occupational Therapy Services

Occupational therapy addresses a person's needs and desires to participate in meaningful activities in their lives. The occupational therapy profession addresses three aspects of performance: the daily life activities that the person wants and needs to do (i.e., performance areas), a person's skills to perform (i.e., performance components), and the environments in which persons perform their daily life tasks (i.e., performance contexts). Tables 6-1, 6-2 and 6-3 present lists of the performance areas, performance components, and performance contexts addressed by the occupational therapist.

There are three core principles that underlie the occupational therapy service provision process. First, occupational therapists consider the person's and the family's desired outcomes and the relationships among these outcomes and current performance. Second, they consider the relevant contexts for desired outcomes. Third, occupational therapists identify appropriate collaborators to design pertinent methods of intervention to support the person and family as they work toward desired functional outcomes. Each of these is discussed separately.

Needs Are Related to Desired Outcomes

When persons cannot perform their daily life tasks as identified in Table 6-1, occupational therapy professionals analyze how persons attempt to perform the tasks to figure out what might be helping or creating barriers to performance. The occupational therapist uses skilled observation, interview/history-taking, records review, and formal and informal assessment to obtain pertinent information. The occupational therapist always keeps a focus on the desired performance outcome, because performance in daily life is the primary concern of occupational therapy services.

Table 6-1
PERFORMANCE AREAS ADDRESSED IN OCCUPATIONAL THERAPY

Performance Areas: Necessary or desired life tasks

Activities of Daily Living	*Work and Productive Activities*	*Play or Leisure Activities*
1. Grooming	1. Home Management	1. Play or Leisure Exploration
2. Oral Hygiene	a. Clothing Care	2. Play or Leisure Performance
3. Bathing/Showering	b. Cleaning	
4. Toilet Hygiene	c. Meal Preparation/Cleanup	
5. Personal Device Care	d. Shopping	
6. Dressing	e. Money Management	
7. Feeding and Eating	f. Household Maintenance	
8. Medication Routine	g. Safety Procedures	
9. Health Maintenance	2. Care of Others	
10. Socialization	3. Educational Activities	
11. Functional Communication	4. Vocational Activities	
12. Functional Mobility	a. Vocational Exploration	
13. Community Mobility	b. Job Acquisition	
14. Emergency Response	c. Work or Job Performance	
15. Sexual Expression	d. Retirement Planning	
	e. Volunteer Participation	

From: American Occupational Therapy Association, Inc. (1994). *Uniform Terminology for Occupational Therapy* (3rd ed.). Rockville, MD: Author.

Table 6-2 presents the list of performance components the occupational therapist considers during this process. Occupational therapists consider specific performance component deficits based on Table 6-2 only if they interfere with the person's ability to perform necessary or desired life tasks. For example, if the family of a child with difficulty solving problems had a goal for the child to develop social skills with peers, the team could select socialization activities that would emphasize sensorimotor skills and minimize the use of cognitive skills, so that the child could have successful play experiences. Examples of service provision options are presented in Table 6.3.

Table 6-2
PERFORMANCE COMPONENTS ADDRESSED IN OCCUPATIONAL THERAPY

Sensorimotor Component	*Cognitive Integration and Cognitive Component*	*Psychosocial Skills and Psychological Components*
1. Sensory	1. Level of Arousal	1. Psychological
a. Sensory Awareness	2. Orientation	a. Values
b. Sensory Processing	3. Recognition	b. Interests
1. Tactile	4. Attention Span	c. Self-Concept
2. Proprioceptive	5. Initiation of Activity	2. Social
3. Vestibular	6. Termination of Activity	a. Role Performance
4. Visual	7. Memory	b. Social Conduct
5. Auditory	8. Sequencing	c. Interpersonal Skills
6. Gustatory	9. Categorization	d. Self-Expression
7. Olfactory	10. Concept Formation	3. Self-Management
c. Perceptual Skills	11. Spatial Operations	a. Coping
1. Stereognosis	12. Problem Solving	b. Time Management
2. Kinesthesia	13. Learning	c. Self-Control
3. Pain Response	14. Generalization	
4. Body Scheme		
5. Right-Left Discrimination		
6. Form Constancy		
7. Position in Space		
8. Visual Closure		
9. Figure-Ground		
10. Depth Perception		
11. Spatial Relations		
12. Topographical Orientation		
2. Neuromuscular		
a. Reflex		
b. Range of Motion		
c. Muscle Tone		
d. Strength		
e. Endurance		
f. Postural Control		
g. Postural Alignment		
h. Soft tissue Integrity		

3. Motor
   a. Gross Coordination
   b. Crossing the Midline
   c. Laterality
   d. Bilateral Integration
   e. Motor Control
   f. Praxis
   g. Fine Coordination/Dexterity
   h. Visual-Motor Integration
   i. Oral-Motor Control

From: American Occupational Therapy Association, Inc. (1994). *Uniform Terminology for Occupational Therapy* (3rd ed.). Rockville, MD: Author.

Table 6-3
EXAMPLES OF SERVICE PROVISION OPTIONS
WHEN CONSIDERING MODELS AND APPROACHES TOGETHER

SERVICE PROVISION APPROACHES

SERVICE PROVISION MODELS	ESTABLISH/ RESTORE (remediate)	ADAPT (compensate)	ALTER	PREVENT	CREATE (promote)
DIRECT	facilitate neck extensor muscle so child can look at friends when playing	fabricate a splint to enable the child to hold the cup at snack time	select a community preschool based on the level of noise the child can manage	facilitate weight bearing during infancy to prevent possible delays in walking	provide a play program for the community for all children to attend
MONITORING	supervise the teacher's aide to facilitate tone for reaching during a game	supervise a feeding program which minimizes the time for eating, and enables socialization	work with parents to identify which community locations will be best for their family outings	create a "positions alternatives" chart for the aides to prevent skin breakdowns	oversee the develop-ment of a morning preschool routine that optimizes early develop-ment possiblities

CONSULTATION	teach classroom staff how to incorporate enhanced sensory input into play routines during free time	show teachers how to change the piece of a game so all children can handle the pieces	provide team with information from skilled observations which enable them to select the best play partner for a child	teach parent a range of motion sequence to prevent deformities	assist the day care provider to develop a compre-hensive curriculum

From: Dunn, W. (1998). Occupational Therapy. In McWilliams, R. (Ed.). *Integrated Services in Center-Based Early Intervention.*

Desired Outcomes Must Occur in Relevant Contexts

It makes a big difference where persons perform daily life tasks (Dunn, Brown, & McGuigan, 1994). Washing your hands at home or in the sink at the back of a classroom can make a difference because each sink area is like-ly to be set up differently. If a young child has learned the routine at home, it may be confusing to find the soap and towels in the classroom sink area. If the baby sitter's home is too noisy, the baby may not be able to get to sleep; changing the context by moving the baby to a more isolated part of the house might help the baby sleep.

Contexts are not just the physical areas in which we perform tasks; con-texts also include the persons, their reactions and expectations (i.e., social and cultural contexts), and their age, stage of disability, and other temporal features of context. The occupational therapist thinks about how the context might be contributing to, or interfering with, the person's performance. The occupational therapist uses this information to determine whether the con-text needs to be adapted for the person and family, or whether the person can improve sensorimotor, cognitive, or psychosocial skills to manage the context more successfully (Dunn, 1990). Many times both strategies are use-ful.

Occupational therapists prioritize using natural contexts for interventions, because they are filled with inherent properties that support functional behavior. For instance, the bathroom contains sinks, which may remind us to wash our hands; the preschool has peers who respond spontaneously to a child's actions. When interventions support children to acquire skills in nat-ural environments, these environments can provide cues and supports for the behavior throughout the day (Dunn, 1996).

Collaboration Enhances Our Ability to Produce Functional Outcomes

Occupational therapists consider what persons and their families want or need to do in their lives. Joining with others in the collaborative process of problem-solving produces more effective interventions. Other professionals and family members and the occupational therapist have complementary perspectives on a particular situation. Occupational therapists value others' viewpoints as an important part of creating an optimal intervention plan. The occupational therapist can create intervention plans that fit into the person's lifestyle and life contexts when other key people provide information. Collaboration enables the team to create interventions which incorporate all facets of the individual's needs into the life routines (Dunn, in press; Idol, Paolucci-Whitcomb & Nevin, 1987).

Relationship to Other Disciplines

Occupational therapy emphasizes children's functional abilities as they seek to perform life tasks that are important to them and their families. This emphasis complements other disciplines, highlighting the importance of the interdisciplinary team. Table 6-4 summarizes the overlap between occupational therapy and several other disciplines, and provides an example of strategies which can be used to coordinate services. This table does not provide a comprehensive analysis but rather a sample of key areas of interest as these professions collaborate on teams (Dunn, 1993).

Table 6-4
RELATIONSHIP BETWEEN OCCUPATIONAL THERAPY AND
OTHER DISCIPLINES
Strategies for Coordinating Services

DISCIPLINE	OVERLAP WITH OCCUPATIONAL THERAPY	STRATEGIES FOR COORDINATION OF SERVICES
Physical Therapy	understanding the human body and its function and capacities; understanding the developmental process across the life span	PT can provide preparatory work to increase tolerance/ capacity for activity; OT can apply the capacities to the desired functional task;
Social Work	recognition of the importance of individuals living and working in the community; understanding the importance of family supports	SW can provide specific links to the community for the family, and can facilitate movement through the systems to obtain desired resources and placements

		when needed; OT prepares the child and family to function within desired settings
Special Education	understanding the cognitive aspects of performance; understanding task analysis	SPED can provide the cognitive tasks that are appropriate for the child; OT considers the sensori-motor, cognitive, and psychosocial aspects of the particular cognitive tasks; they collaborate to create a single intervention
Speech Language Pathology	knowledge of the oral motor structures; knowledge of the swallow patterns; knowledge of the non-verbal aspects of communication	SP can provide swallowing interventions; OT can address food acquisition and oral motor control; SP can provide expertise regarding the selection of the proper augmentative communication device; OT addresses functional aspects of communication device; OT addresses functional aspects of communication, e.g., access to augmentative devices

From: Dunn, W. (1992). Occupational Therapy Evaluation. In: F.R. Brown, E.H. Aylward, and B.K. Keogh (Eds.), *Diagnosis and Management of Learning Disabilities: An Interdisciplinary/Lifestyle* (2nd ed.) San Diego: Singular Publishing Group, Inc.

CONTRIBUTIONS OF OCCUPATIONAL THERAPY TO INTERDISCIPLINARY PRACTICE

The occupational therapy profession emphasizes the child's performance of daily life tasks. To accomplish this emphasis, occupational therapy personnel have the expertise to analyze tasks, assess the child's skills, and identify the supports and barriers in the context. They are interested in the meaning the child and family derive from the daily life tasks they prioritize. Interventions that include occupational therapists will address functional outcomes within the context of daily life.

Key Issues Regarding Participation on Teams

All team members face challenges as they collaborate. Team members must value other perspectives by believing that one point of view is unacceptable in creating optimal plans. Since traditional higher education programs have taught most professionals in isolation from other disciplines, this perspective is sometimes difficult for professionals to embrace.

In discussing how educator/therapist partnerships emerge, Matter and Weinstein (1988) state that teachers have found the medical model approach of programming to be foreign to them, while therapists were unfamiliar with curriculum design, making it difficult to relate therapy concerns to classroom activities. As therapists began to understand the curricula, they began to offer suggestions for the curriculum that were improvements for all the children. Teachers became more aware of the individual differences that might affect school activities. These insights on both partners' parts enabled new schemas to emerge for assessing children, with combined emphases on individual skills and functional performance in school.

Everyone is a winner when the intervention plan fits the family's lifestyle, the child's learning or play preferences, and when it addresses key functional needs and desires. Everyone loses when one discipline dominates unnecessarily, causing the solution to have the appearance of that discipline, rather than the family and the child's lifestyle (Dunn, 1996).

Team members must believe that the child's and family's needs are more important than the visibility of their own discipline. Sometimes a member of one discipline needs to retract a recommendation because it is not consistent with the child and family's needs and interests. For example, the occupational therapist may identify serious oral motor problems which will interfere with talking and eating. However, oral motor intervention for talking would not be appropriate if the team determined that an augmentative communication device was a better option. The occupational therapist might work on reaching and pointing skills needed to gain access to the device for communication.

It is critical that collaborative programming embrace equal partnerships among team members. Group leadership can be flexible to meet family needs. Collaborators also recognize the importance of having other team members present in addition to their reports during meetings; more flexible scheduling ensures that critical points of view are represented (Rainforth, York, & MacDonald, 1993). Idol et al. (1987) provide a benchmark discussion of the principles of collaborative consultation and provide methods for developing these skills.

Teamwork requires professionals to focus on other adults (i.e., parents and other professionals) who don't give us the same direct, concrete feedback as children do. Team members must learn how to give each other reinforcement for work well done.

Concepts of Integrating Services

The concept of integrating therapeutic interventions into natural environments and daily tasks is not new to the related service disciplines (Dunn, Moore, Brown, & Westman, 1994), although its implementation has been slow to occur. For example, the philosophical constructs of occupational therapy are based on the concept of purposeful activity or those tasks that have meaning for the individual, because meaningfulness provides intrinsic motivation to persist in reaching goals (Breines, 1984; Clark, 1979; Fidler & Fidler, 1978; Hinojosa, Sabari, Rosenfeld, & Shapiro, 1983; Kircher, 1984; West, 1984; Steinbeck, 1986). Kircher (1984) and Steinbeck (1986) both found that persons without disabilities persisted significantly longer on an identical task of exertion when the task had an identifiable purpose, rather than when perceived merely as an exercise. Gliner (1985) proposed that professionals create typical life events for learning motor skills, suggesting that the person and environment are inseparable.

Giangreco, Edelman, and Dennis (1991) studied professional practices that facilitate or interfere with integrated services. Writing individual discipline goals, recommendations, and reports before meetings and making placement decisions based on available services rather than the child's needs interfere with integrated programming. They recommend group goal and recommendation development, with an emphasis on the children's needs and strengths, rather than those that are associated with a particular discipline.

Positive outcomes can occur for children when professionals implement newer models of service provision. Dunn (1990) compared direct intervention and consultation in preschool programs for children with developmental delays. Although both service provision models yielded the same percentage of IEP goals being met (approximately 70 percent) when teachers collaborated in a consultation model, they reported that the occupational therapist contributed effort to 24 percent more of the goals on the IEP. Peck, Killen and Baumgart (1989) demonstrated that consultation encouraged teachers to develop effective interventions on simple language goals for children with disabilities. Additionally, teachers generalized the techniques to new situations that were not part of the initial project. Giangreco (1986) compared isolated therapy services with integrated occupational and physical therapy services (i.e., teacher and therapists collaborate to design the intervention) for a student with multiple disabilities. The student performed significantly better during the integrated intervention phase, supporting the effectiveness of integrating teacher and therapist expertise. Jones (1983) combined several therapy techniques with behavioral techniques to investigate eating problems in children with mental retardation. Combined approaches were most effective at supporting the children to eat solid foods. The related service literature contains clear indications that integrating the ideas from several disciplines can be an effective means of servicing children with disabilities and their families.

THE ROLES PARENTS TYPICALLY PLAY IN THE OPTIMAL INTERDISCIPLINARY SERVICE PROVISION OF OCCUPATIONAL THERAPY

Parents are critical collaborators for occupational therapy personnel, because they are the ones (along with their children, when that is possible) who determine the focus of assessment and intervention. Since occupational therapists are concerned with performance in daily life, it is imperative that they know what daily life tasks are important and necessary to those who are seeking their support. With younger children, the family is the only source of accurate information; with older children, the family and school personnel are the most common sources of information.

The family's input frames the entire assessment and intervention process for occupational therapy. Although the occupational therapist may identify difficulties in a wide range of performance areas, only those difficulties that impact the tasks of interest to the family are addressed in intervention.

Families must also provide feedback to the occupational therapist about the child's performance at home during intervention because this is the true test of the success of the intervention. It is not appropriate to judge the success of interventions by measuring components such as balance, without finding out how the child's balance improvements are affecting daily life tasks. For example, if the child's standardized score for balance increases, but the child continues to have difficulty getting clothing and toys out of the closet, the occupational therapist's goals would not be met.

TYPICAL PARENT QUESTIONS/COMMENTS FOR OCCUPATIONAL THERAPISTS

What is sensory integration therapy, and how does it work?

Sensory integration is a theory about how sensory input, information processing and movement planning affect the child's performance. It is a way of thinking about the meaning of the child's responses to events in daily life. Like other theories, sensory integration does not answer all the questions about performance but rather provides another way to look at the child's activity. It helps professionals gain a different insight into current skills and possible methods for supporting the child to function better in the environment.

Sensory integration is based on the premise that human beings take in sensory information, interpret this information, and then create a response. The neuroscience literature is rich with information about how these processes operate. A. Jean Ayres and others have developed an application of this neuroscience knowledge as they have hypothesized how behavior reflects these operations. Some authors have criticized the use of sensory integration (e.g., Arendt, MacLean, & Baumeister, 1988), while others have demonstrated its usefulness (see Fisher, Bundy, & Murray, 1991). Newer diagnostic information about children with various disabilities (e.g., autism, ADHD, regulatory disorders) acknowledges the role of sensory processing in the performance patterns of these children (National Center for Clinical Infant Programs, 1994). What is important are the neuroscience principles upon which the sensory integration theory is based. Active research programs continue to reveal knowledge about sensory integration and its application to practice.

Sensory integration is core knowledge from the occupational therapy profession, and so it is appropriate to expect occupational therapists on your teams to be knowledgeable about this theory. Other team members may acquire this knowledge from continuing education or graduate school experiences. It is important to remember that sensory integration is a frame of reference for the professional's thinking. Professionals are not "sensory integration therapists;" they are occupational therapists who can use this theory in their work.

When using sensory integration as part of assessment and intervention planning, the therapist will consider the sensory processing feature of performance. For example, if dressing were the concern, the occupational therapist would want to know about the textures of clothing (including looseness or snugness, as in elastic), because different textures send different messages to the brain. Some children pull on tags, or are very rigid about what types of socks and underwear they will wear. The occupational therapist would hypothesize that the way these items feel on the skin could be contributing to the child's disruptive behaviors because they keep the child focused on the items (e.g., ripping at the tags, fidgeting in the chair, shuffling the feet), and make it difficult to concentrate on other tasks. The therapist would work with the parents to identify what makes certain items troublesome and offer alternatives that would reduce these interfering behaviors (i.e., the child would be more comfortable and would be able to move on).

Sensory integration traditionally has been used in isolated direct services, but more and more commonly therapists and teams are incorporating sensory integration principles into daily routines at school and home. Levels of noise, the amount of visual stimuli, amounts of movement in routines, and being touched during tasks can all affect performance. Dealing with these factors in the natural course of living provides many more opportunities for a therapeutic event than having only isolated treatment for sensory processing needs. Although some children may need specialized services in a less distracting and more focused environment, applying sensory integration principles to the routines of the day capitalizes on this theory's impact on children's lives.

My daughter is three years old and she sees her OT twice weekly. The OT gives us home activities for my child, but we rarely get around to doing them given the other demands of our home. I feel guilty. Do you have advice about how we can increase our participation in our child's therapy in a family friendly way?

When professionals work with families they have an obligation to provide expertise and support as part of the family's way of life. In your situation, you and the therapist must begin to act like you are equal partners in the endeavor of serving your child and family. This means that the therapist must find out what your lifestyle is like so that home suggestions are compatible with your life routine. As equal members of this team, you must speak up about your needs and constraints (e.g., time, resources, routines) and not allow your team (i.e., you and your provider) to design a home program that is incompatible with your life. The only effective home suggestions are those that: (1) fit into the routines, because these are the only ones that get implemented anyway; and (2) support family members to bond with each other as a family, not as substitute therapists doing therapy.

The knowledge and expertise of an occupational therapist is well suited to making your daily routines therapeutic events, rather than disrupting your life to find time for therapy. For example, when children need their diapers changed, there are opportunities for eye contact, verbal and social interactions, increasing flexibility in joints and muscles, providing sensory input to increase body awareness, and hand play to improve eye-hand coordination. Therapists can guide the parent through diapering, pointing out what to do while completing this family routine. While on the back, your child doesn't have to work so hard to keep the head and body upright, so this frees up energy to look around, watch your face, and move hands into view. Being on the back also makes it easier for the legs to open up, so playing with the child's legs to encourage this flexibility is therapeutic. You don't have to set up a separate therapy time to lay on the floor and stretch or have hand play time.

Whenever parents begin to feel guilty, there is a tendency to withhold information from the therapist, fearing that the therapist will judge them as bad or uncaring parents. If your therapist does this, get a new one; an insightful and family-centered therapist will feel badly for having suggested items that weren't compatible for you, and will want to immediately proceed to collaborating on a new plan. But remember, this is also your responsibility as a collaborator to speak up so your needs are addressed; professionals cannot read minds. Suggestions that are good for one family will not be suitable for another, and the only informant about this is the child and family.

Dr. Schulz's Response:

The author's response is right on target in emphasizing that home activities be relevant and meaningful to the home situation. Even so, it may be difficult for busy parents to integrate the home activities prescribed by the therapist.

Siblings and extended family members can be involved in the home activities, learning new skills themselves and becoming important members on the team. There are several principles to remember in using these valuable resources. First, they do need to be trained, either by the therapist or by the parents who have been instructed in specific processes. Second, the experience needs to be rewarding for them and not become an unwelcome burden. For example, siblings could take turns with the activities, relinquishing a household duty for the time needed. With extended family members a gift, a meal, or a simple thank-you may be rewarding. Ultimately, the progress of the child with the disability is both the goal and the reward.

Our son sees an OT and a PT. It looks like a lot of the same things are happening in each session. How do these two types of therapies differ, and how are they alike?

I would first want to know how old your son is, what his performance needs are and the setting for therapy in order to respond specifically to your experience. However, there are some general issues that are relevant within your question.

Both occupational therapy and physical therapy training include an in-depth analysis of how persons move and control themselves with respect to gravity. Both professions have expertise in the ways that movement affects performance. It is common in children's services for one of the disciplines to see the children and use the other discipline to provide support. For example, physical therapy is more likely to take the lead with locomotion issues, sitting postures and balance problems, while an occupational therapist is more likely to take the lead when the referral problems are related to daily life, such as dressing, eating and socialization. In both cases, however, the other discipline's knowledge will come into play. When the physical therapist is working on balance, she might be concerned how that balance is affecting lunch time and ask for occupational therapy support for this aspect of treatment. When the occupational therapist is working on dressing and eating, he might call on the physical therapist to look at trunk alignment and support (i.e., holding the body and head up) during this task.

There are distinct differences between occupational therapy and physical therapy services. Physical therapists are more interested in the person's physical capacity and its relation to performance, while occupational therapists use their knowledge about the person's abilities and limitations to examine how the person conducts daily life activities. The occupational therapist's interest is in the ways that the person can (or cannot) do the things the person wants and needs to do in daily life (i.e., the intersection between the person, the task the person wishes to perform, and the environment in which the person conducts daily life). Physical therapy is more likely to use exercise as a modality in treatment, while occupational therapy is more likely to use activities as the treatment modality.

Young children spend a lot of their time playing. Because of this method of interacting, it is not surprising to see occupational therapy and physical therapy looking the same. With their respective interests in movement and activity, play is a great and compatible medium for therapy. However, parents have the responsibility to ask what the goals are in these sessions to be sure that their family's goals are addressed. Therapists cannot presume that anyone is going to address family needs without the family raising the appropriate issues and concerns. Children only learn to dress themselves with guidance and support; children with disabilities need supports to learn many schemas, even playing patterns. So it is not appropriate for therapists to conduct therapy without clearly and directly addressing the tasks and goals for the family. Children will not automatically generalize their balance skills to new tasks without support from family and therapists. If therapists look like their work is the same, ask the question why your child needs to have two therapists for these activities when there are so many skills to address. It is more common for therapists to work in concert with the family and teachers to design therapeutic activities throughout the child's day. Then the team takes responsibility for generalizing new skills to actual performance situations.

I was surprised to find an OT on my child's feeding team. What are the OT's contributions to feeding with young children?

As you have learned in this chapter, occupational therapists focus on performance in daily life. Feeding and eating are central to daily routines, and therefore the interdisciplinary team frequently seeks out occupational therapy expertise to ensure they are considering the feeding issues comprehensively.

On a feeding team, the occupational therapist will address a number of issues. Children might have difficulty with eating because of sensorimotor, cognitive, or psychosocial issues (person issues); might need support in learning eating routines (task issues); or might need particular environmental supports to eat successfully (context issues).

As part of a feeding evaluation team, the occupational therapist might assess the child's awareness of or sensitivity to various food textures and temperatures, and record the way the child uses the lips, tongue, teeth, and palate to move food through the mouth. The occupational therapist would watch the ways that the child approaches the task of eating, such as hand-to-mouth movements, leaning over the food, to see if any of these actions are ineffective. If the parent feeds the child, the interaction between them in negotiating eating would be of interest. For example, the child might have a better time swallowing if the parent holds the child in a new position, or if they use a different utensil. The occupational therapist would also want to know about environmental variables, such as the meal time routine for the family, the chairs, whether the TV is on during meals, and the time schedules for eating. All of these factors can support or be disruptive to the process of eating. The occupational therapist would analyze the impact of person, task, and context variables to make recommendations to the team and family.

CASE EXAMPLE

Alicia is a four-year-old who attends a community preschool and daycare program. Alicia does fine during free play periods and seems to enjoy small group, teacher-directed activities, but Alicia is very disruptive and unsuccessful during snack times. Parents report that Alicia does fine at meal times at home, commenting that they prepare her foods so she will eat them, provide a very structured ritual, and they believe Alicia can concentrate on the business of eating since it is just she and her parents at the table.

The team decided that the assessment ought to include a skilled observation of snack time and a more in-depth interview of the parents about meal time rituals. The occupational therapist and the preschool teacher conducted the skilled observation, and the occupational therapist interviewed the parents and collected sensory history data from them.

The sensory history revealed some possible reasons why snack time was difficult for Alicia. Alicia had difficulty with auditory, touch, oral and multisensory processing. The parent interview revealed that Alicia's parents have been very intuitive. They minimized the impact of particular aspects of the eating experience that had proven to be difficult. For example, they created a quieter, less auditorily challenging environment during meal time (e.g., no

TV or radio on). They prepared foods Alicia liked, and have not challenged her limited range of food interests.

The day care center staff had bigger challenges. During the skilled observation, the teacher and the therapist identified several issues. With eight children at the table, snack time was much more unpredictable. The daycare staff introduced tastes and textures that Alicia was unfamiliar with, making her sense of discomfort with the situation more apparent. With poor ability to process touch stimuli, and oral sensitivity to textures and tastes as is indicated on the sensory history from the parents, snack time was providing a combination of stimuli which exceeded Alicia's thresholds. The therapist and teacher also discussed the possibility that Alicia's internal control skills were undeveloped, since she performed better when parents were controlling the situation. The therapist made a note to include the behavior specialist in their discussions to investigate behavior management strategies that might complement the overall intervention plan.

The team was also concerned about Alicia's disruptive behavior. While other children are also active about interacting in their environments in the preschool years, they learn and profit from these interactions. Alicia may have been attempting to engage in her environment, but with her difficulties in processing certain types of sensory information, her attempts led to disruptions for both herself and her peers.

The team was anxious for the parents to share strategies about meal time. The team discussed their perceptions about the differences in Alicia's performance from home to school and brainstormed with the parents about how to help Alicia be successful.

In a situation such as this, understanding the parameters of performance in different settings becomes important to interpretation and intervention planning. Without having formal training, Alicia's parents had intuitively provided what she needed. This action had minimized the effects of her poor sensory processing on her performance at home. The challenge in serving children like Alicia is that the team must balance between providing supports to enable successful performance and providing opportunities to experience sensory input and modulation successfully. A good rule of thumb is to provide supports for sensory processing problems during more difficult tasks while designing other opportunities for the child to receive and process sensory input. Professionals must not act on the outdated idea that because Alicia is young, intervention must focus on learning how to deal with things.

For Alicia, her troubles at snack time occurred because this activity required modulation of all the sensory inputs that are the most challenging for her. If nutrition or her disruptive behavior are extreme barriers, the team would initiate adaptive strategies during snack time. For example, to reduce the chances of others bumping into Alicia, the teacher could place her at the end of the table (thereby reducing tactile opportunities). Ear plugs or muffs dampen the effect of ambient noise during snack time. Team members would need to try several adaptations to find out what worked for Alicia, because with poor tactile processing, furry muffs or tight plugs might be irritating. Since Alicia is four years old, ear muffs with animal heads might be appealing. By tapping the parents' expertise, the team can prepare snacks that are within Alicia's oral sensory tolerances, to reduce her outbursts from the unpleasant sensations in her mouth.

At other times during the preschool day, the team might design sensory processing opportunities to help Alicia develop more adaptability. For example, mouth play (e.g., blowing, sucking, and making faces in the mirror), and self-care routines such as face washing can provide opportunities for Alicia to develop oral sensory awareness. The family can build on their successful routine to slowly introduce new textures and tastes into her diet at home. They can also introduce background music, noticing which sounds (e.g., talking, classical, country) are easier for her to manage. At the day care center, they can work in groups at the table separate from eating, incorporating auditory and tactile experiences into the activities (e.g., finger painting, singing, and clapping). In these ways, Alicia has opportunities to successfully process sensory input for successful performance.

Outcomes from Team Planning

When the teachers introduced the ear muffs, Alicia kept pulling them off. At first, everyone thought she hated the muffs, but the day care provider noticed that Alicia was not throwing them away. Rather, she was taking them off and then looking at the animal faces. So the teachers decided to teach Alicia to look in the mirror to see the puppies, and they posted a picture of her wearing the puppy ear muffs by the snack table. These strategies stopped Alicia from removing the muffs, and she wore them during the snack time ritual.

The therapist was very impressed by their ability to analyze Alicia's overall behaviors and not jump to the wrong conclusion in their frustration to find better snack time strategies. The muffs did seem to help with extra noise at snack time, and sometimes Alicia would wear them to play outside as well.

Introducing new textures was a little harder. Alicia continued to be very resistant, but with experimentation the teachers identified several strategies. For example, when foods were a more neutral temperature, Alicia was more likely to accept a new texture (e.g., warm apple sauce rather than cold apple sauce). She also responded well to a cognitive approach (i.e., the teachers asked the children which food was softer, e.g., pudding) or harder (e.g., cookie). Under these conditions, Alicia would join in with the other children more readily.

What was important to the teachers was understanding the parameters of Alicia's difficulty. This knowledge helped them to be more accurate observers and to make adjustments within the proper parameters for Alicia's needs.

Editors' Note:

Dunn does an excellent job of describing and promoting family-centered practices. Regardless of the team model selected, families must drive decision-making. For many professionals, this will mean learning new ways to conduct business. We believe the effort will be worth the return as families become empowered partners in the service delivery process.

REFERENCES

Arendt, R. E., MacLean, W. E., Jr. and Baumeister, A. A. (1988). Critique of sensory integration therapy and its application in mental retardation. *American Journal of Mental Retardation 92*, 401-411.

Breines, E. (1984). An attempt to define purposeful activity. *American Journal of Occupational Therapy, 38*, 543-544.

Clark, P. N. (1979). Human development through occupation: Theoretical frameworks in contemporary occupational therapy practice, Part 1. *American Journal of Occupational Therapy, 33*, 505-514.

Dunn, W. (1990). A comparison of service provision models in school-based occupational therapy services. *American Journal of Occupational Therapy.*

Dunn, W. (1996). Occupational Therapy. In R. A. McWilliams (Ed.), *Rethinking pullout services in early intervention: A professional resource* (267-314). Baltimore: MD: Paul H. Brookes.

Dunn, W. (in press). Person centered and contextually relevant evaluation. In J. Hinojosa & P. Kramer (Eds.), *Occupational therapy evaluation: Obtaining and interpreting data.* Bethesda, MD: American Occupational Therapy Association.

Dunn, W., Brown, C., & McGuigan, A. (1994). The ecology of human performance: A framework for considering the effect of context. *American Journal of Occupational Therapy, 48*, 595-607.

Dunn, W., Moore, W., Brown, C. & Westman, K. (1994). Development of a consolidated model for providing inclusive education and related services for children and youth with disabilities. Unfunded OSEP Grant.

Fidler, G. S., & Fidler, J. W. (1978). Doing and becoming: Purposeful action and self actualization. *American Journal of Occupational Therapy, 32*, 305-310.

Fisher, A., Bundy, A., and Murray, E. (1991). *Sensory integration.* Philadelphia: F.A. Davis.

Giangreco, M. F., Edelman, S., & Dennis, R. (1991). Common professional practices that interfere with the integrated delivery of related services. *Remdial and Special Education, 12,* 16-24.

Hinojosa, J., Sabari, J., Rosenfeld, M. S., & Shapiro, M. S. (1983). Purposeful activities. *American Journal of Occupational Therapy, 37,* 805-806.

Idol, L., Paolucci-Whitcomb, P., & Nevin, A. (1987). *Collaborative consultation.* Austin, TX: Pro-Ed.

Kircher, M. A. (184). Motivation as a factor of perceived exertion in purposeful versus nonpurposeful activity. *American Journal of Occupational Therapy, 38,* 165-170.

National Center for Clinical Infant Programs. (1994). *Diagnostic Classification of Mental Health and Development Disorders of Infancy and Early Childhood.*

Rainforth, B., MacDonald, C., & York, J. (1993). Collaborative teamwork: Integrated therapy services in educational programs for students with severe disabilities. Baltimore: Paul H. Brookes.

Steinbeck, T. N. (1986). Purposeful activity and performance. *American Journal of Occupational Therapy, 40,* 529-534.

West, W. L. (1984). A reaffirmed philosophy and practice of occupational therapy for the 1980s. *American Journal of Occupational Therapy, 38,* 15-23.

Chapter 7

PHYSICAL THERAPY

KATHERINE LEGUIN WHITE

Physical therapy in the United States was spawned during World War I. Concerned about the physical well-being of wounded soldiers, the Surgeon General instituted training programs and hospital clinics to create a corps of reconstruction aides. Miss Mary McMillian was recruited to develop their training program. An American who had studied physical therapy in England prior to the war, Miss McMillian was working in a London orthopedic surgeon's office when the war broke out. Responding to the Surgeon General's request, she returned home in 1918 to teach reconstruction aides at Reed College in Portland, Oregon. Then and there American physical therapy was born (Murphy, 1995).

Later in the century, when America was plagued with continuous, persistent epidemics of polio, physical therapists again worked with orthopedists, neurosurgeons, and neurologists to respond to a national need. This time they came to help relieve pain and restore function to thousands of children and adults who had contracted polio.

During both national crises, physical therapists, working closely with physicians, became proficient in the use of physical agents. They used therapeutic exercise, hydrotherapy, heat, electricity, and massage to help individual patients regain function of their arms and legs or adjust physically to a loss of function. Emphasis on physical function and physical therapeutic methods was the original and, hence, traditional focus of physical therapy practice.

The heritage/history of physical therapy, therefore, was individual patient care organized around therapeutic applications of physical agents and fidelity to principles of the medical model of care. Physical therapists used cause and effect rationales, specific treatments for specific injuries or illnesses with individual patient-therapist relationships. Medical practice during the 1930s and 1940s guided the education and practice of physical therapists in the United States during the early twentieth century.

Other simultaneous influences in the early development of physical therapy came from physical education, physical culture movements, and the evolving profession of rehabilitation medicine or physiatry (Grover, 1989). Gradually, after both world wars, physicians and physical therapists expanded their practices to embrace concerns for the lifelong implications of physical injury and illness.

MAJOR ROLES AND RESPONSIBILITIES OF PHYSICAL THERAPISTS

Today, all fifty states have licensure laws that govern physical therapy practice. One prerequisite for licensure is graduation from an accredited education program for physical therapists. While the medical model of treatment continues to dominate many physical therapy education curricula, alternate educational models are gaining attention. These focus on patient function, collaboration with families and professional colleagues, and therapeutic interventions embodying psychosocial, political, and economic as well as physical principles.

Today, few physical therapists practice in doctors' offices. Many physical therapists now practice in acute and tertiary care settings. However, they also practice increasingly in elementary and secondary schools, state and local health departments, daycare and sheltered employment programs, long-term care facilities, interdisciplinary and multispecialty clinics, and in patients' homes. Physical therapy educators increasingly structure curricula around the dynamics of primary care and interdisciplinary practice in preference over traditional medical rehabilitation and individual treatment models.

Another role practiced more frequently by physical therapists is that of primary care provider. Licensure laws in thirty-nine states provide authority for therapists to accept patients directly without having first been referred by a physician. The specific requirements of this so-called direct access legislation vary from state to state. It generally means, however, that physical therapists may at least evaluate patients without previous medical treatment and/or referral. It is advisable for parents to check their state boards of physical therapy licensure to determine whether they need a physician's referral for physical therapy.

As physical therapy practice becomes more scientific, it is also more collaborative and concentrated on patients' functional outcomes instead of application of physical agents. Today, therapeutic exercises and play therapy are most frequently used by physical therapists who work with children and adults with developmental disabilities. Ice and heat continue to be used, however, to reduce pain and muscle tone, and to enhance the effects of exercise. Therapeutic use of exercise has become the preferred approach of physical therapists as scientists better understand and increasingly apply motor learning principles to rehabilitation of all disabilities.

Therapeutic exercise for infants and toddlers, school-age children, and teenagers often is accomplished through play activities. Games, toys, puppets, and objects that provide sensory stimulation, such as sand and water, all become vehicles for exercise. Participation in competitive sports through typical and adapted programs helps children and young adults develop coordination, strength, endurance, and balance. Sports also enhance social skills (through team building and teamwork) and participation in family and community life. Exercise, therefore, takes many forms. The challenge for physical therapists is to match the exercise with the special needs of an individual child or adult.

Working teenagers and adults who are developmentally disabled may have unique physical therapy needs in their places of employment. Physical therapists can help these individuals organize their work spaces, maintain physical fitness for efficient and effective use of their bodies, and prevent injuries in the work place. Physical therapists provide consultation to workers with disabilities and their employers. They provide assessment of work environments considering conditions and practices that produce physical trauma or emotional distractions and impediments to optimal performance. Analysis of essential job performance, physical motions, and recommendations for improved work space arrangement can reduce illness or injury caused by repetitive motion.

Individuals with developmental disabilities who approach adulthood have special needs for physical therapy services. Preparation for employment, for life away from home and family, and for participation in community affairs can be enhanced by development of healthy life styles. Physical therapists help in two important ways. First, they assess an individual's physical capacity to perform specific employment tasks and achieve self-sufficiency for individual fitness needs. Second, physical therapists use their assessments to create plans for functional self-sufficiency and continued productive lives into middle age and retirement.

Two frequently discussed definitions of disability emphasize its social dimension. The World Health Organization in 1980 defined disability as "In the context of health experience, a disability is any restriction or lack (resulting from an impairment) of ability to perform an activity in the manner or within the range considered normal for a human being" (p. 28). In 1991, Nagi defined disability as "limitation in performance of such roles and tasks as related to family, work, community, school, recreation within a sociocultural and physical environment" (p. 322). Both definitions point toward relationships with community. Physical therapists enhance communal participation of children and adults with disabilities. Physical therapists now focus their practice on determining the best available treatment for persons with disabilities and how to measure outcomes of those treatments. Many models of functional ability are now being explored by physical therapists. Functional abilities include a wide range of activities from personal care (dressing, feeding, and personal hygiene) to participation in family, employment, and community affairs.

Physical therapists typically concentrate first on assessment of an individual's present functional capacity. For infants and toddlers, functional capacity is measured using normal developmental landmarks such as a child's ability to suck and swallow, to turn from side to side, to sit, stand, and ambulate. Later, a child's ability to dress, to brush his/her teeth, and to eat with a knife and forks is evaluated. And, finally, assessment of a young adult's ability to maintain real or relative independence in self-care and employment or live maximally within the limits of one's disability becomes a major role of physical therapists.

As stated earlier, physical therapy services for children with disabilities most frequently focus on assessment of a child' s musculoskeletal, neurological, and functional capacity. Continuing our profession's faithfulness to the medical model of diagnosis and treatment, physical therapy assessment typically concentrates on gross and fine motor function, muscle tone (rigidity, spasticity, flaccidity), balance, and coordination. Increasingly, physical therapists participate in play-based assessment and arena assessment, replacing emphasis on isolated test parameters, such as physical strength. Physical therapists are increasingly concerned with functional capacities (feeding, toileting, dressing and ambulation) and collaboration with interdisciplinary colleagues.

CONTRIBUTIONS OF PHYSICAL THERAPY TO INTERDISCIPLINARY PRACTICE

Specific contributions of physical therapists to interdisciplinary practice include focused assessment of a child's functional capacities and social interactions that require physical abilities. Physical therapists are not the only health professionals capable of adequately assessing motor learning and function. However, the physical therapy perspective is uniquely important for a thorough determination of a child's or adult's present functional abilities, for predicting a child's future functional attainments, and for realistically focusing a treatment plan at any given point in the life of the child or adult with disabilities.

Frequently it is felt that the contributions of physical therapists and occupational therapists overlap. While this might be true in some particular treatment forums, it is more often true that the two therapists look at the same behavior of a child or adult with different eyes. Physical therapy education still focuses on musculoskeletal and neurological assessment with the aim of improving or increasing a person's physical function. Physical therapy education in the social and behavioral sciences receives less attention than the physical sciences. So physical therapists continue to use physical measures more than those social, cognitive, or psychological assessment and treatment measures in which occupational therapists are more grounded. As physical therapy research advances, physical therapists are becoming more precise in understanding the workings of the central nervous system. Precision and understanding then help physical therapists determine more accurately the origin of a child's motor performance problems and whether there may be a physical therapy remedy for those problems.

Physical and occupational therapists have traditionally been partners in assessment and treatment of children and adults with disabilities. Shared responsibilities, shared insights, and identification of common educational and practice parameters make it easier for occupational therapists and physical therapists to practice collaboratively. All concerned professionals are moving toward collaboration, teamwork, and involvement of patients, families, and communities in search of functional improvement for children and adults with disabilities. Physical therapists are increasingly aware of the need to share their special physical expertise with other team members and families. Physical therapists also are more willing to value other team members' insights, observations, and professional biases and to share their own special talents with colleagues and parents.

Sharing expertise with health professionals and families means that physical therapists must be willing to balance the needs they have identified in a child's or adult's motor performance with the needs identified by families, the child or adult with disabilities, and other health professionals on the team. Joint evaluation and treatment sessions shared with an occupational therapist, a speech-language pathologist, or special education colleague and a parent are more frequently physical therapists' preferred mode of practice. Physical therapists' learned ability to focus sharply on an individual's motor performance becomes one of many perspectives contributed to interdisciplinary practice. Understanding the importance and limits of their expertise helps physical therapists become more effective team members. Accordingly, they sometimes need to sacrifice discipline-specific concerns for a child's physical growth and development to other, more pressing concerns for the child, the child's family, or the community.

When assessing physical function of a child with disabilities, physical therapists are specifically concerned with a child's progress from one developmental landmark to the next. They focus on the child's ability to perform basic functional activities and participate in social interactions, especially those involving motor capacity. Developmental assessment is a shared responsibility that depends as much on the parents' reports of what a child does at home and the observations of other team members as on the specific findings of a physical therapy assessment.

When it comes to basic functional activities, physical therapists and occupational therapists share many of the same professional biases, judgments, and techniques. Nurses and special educators, physicians, and speech-language pathologists are also concerned about a child's functional abilities. Being able to swallow, for example, is a function that concerns many team members, including physical therapists. Each professional brings special knowledge of anatomical and physiological mechanisms involved in the act of swallowing. The physical therapist, for example, is more likely to be concerned with a child's head and trunk posture than with the child's diet or the muscles that are active during swallowing.

Positioning children with disabilities for maximal functioning in numerous activities of daily living is increasingly understood by physical therapists and their colleagues to contribute to speech and language development and improvement. Focus on broad aspects of motor function such as positioning and walking, and ability to operate a wheelchair or other assistive device for ambulation, feeding, or dressing characterizes the physical therapists' role.

Adaptation of equipment and physical environments are also special contributions of physical therapists. From simple things like the kind of bed a child with disabilities sleeps on to more complex technologies, such as computer-assisted movement and learning, physical therapists consult with occupational therapists, rehabilitation engineers, families, and teachers. Physical and occupational therapists often help families rearrange the interiors of their homes to provide easier movement for children in wheelchairs. Physical therapists offer consultation in wheelchair design and construction of ramps to allow persons with disabilities to have increased mobility in their homes and communities.

People often forget that walking is a social function. Physical therapists have traditionally used tests and measurements of musculoskeletal strength, balance, and endurance to analyze a child's ability to walk. Increasingly, they also consider social dimensions of walking. Understanding that walking requires more than muscles and nerves, requires physical therapists to confront several issues. The environment, the people and objects with whom and around whom persons in wheelchairs must maneuver in order to be mobile, and the energy required for children and adults with disabilities to walk are all considerations of the physical therapist.

One of physical therapy's most pressing needs as a profession is learning to collaborate with families, children with disabilities, community, and professional colleagues. The economic and social costs of duplicated efforts and services, conflicting advice and directions, and repetition of tests and interviews previously performed by other evaluators argue for collaboration and coordination of team members. But economic cost alone is not the best reason for collaborating. Increasingly, there is evidence that teamwork is more effective in helping children and their families live good lives. Many researchers and health professionals have believed for decades that quality of care is improved by teamwork. Fortunately, persuasive research by nurses and other health professionals over the past two decades substantiates this belief.

Finally, a major contribution of physical therapists to interdisciplinary practice is education: of children and families about disabilities and how to live good lives with those disabilities, of team members and colleagues about the special vision that physical therapists bring to children and adults with disabilities, to their families, and to their communities.

THE ROLES PARENTS PLAY IN OPTIMAL INTERDISCIPLINARY SERVICE PROVISION OF PHYSICAL THERAPY

Physical therapists benefit greatly from learning about parents' concerns for their children, parents' perceptions of children's functional and social strengths and weaknesses, family routines, and parents' typical daily involvement with their children.

When physical therapists see children during a first assessment session, it is difficult to structure a thorough and true picture of their functional abilities and behaviors from a single assessment session, even when it proceeds smoothly. Not all essential parameters can be evaluated during a one-hour period in a strange place, with one or more unknown persons present to the child. Unable to observe children over the course of a day and night, therapists and other health professionals rely on parents' perceptions of their children's consistent, daily behaviors.

Parents, for example, are often able to elicit behaviors from their children that therapists are not able to stimulate during an evaluation session. Parents may be able to either refute or corroborate a therapist's judgment about a child's specific behavior and the consistency with which the child expresses that behavior. Parents, in this case, help therapists distinguish accidental or splinter behaviors from those consistently and appropriately expressed by a child. In other words, parents are essential for distinguishing real from perceived or misjudged actions a child might demonstrate during an evaluation.

Parents also know a child's limits for responding to focused and requested play or functional activities, and whether a child understands a therapist's directions. Until a therapist has worked with a child long enough to learn what activities or toys elicit a desired behavior, parents are essential for providing this kind of information. A physical therapy evaluation is not complete without parental involvement during the actual physical therapy evaluation and later in a conference. Parents' presence is especially critical to discuss the therapist's observations and whether they conform to a child's daily behavior as observed consistently and over time by a parent or parents.

Parents are also valuable during physical therapy assessment and treatment for their knowledge of how much equipment they can comfortably and safely manage in the home environment. Parents' judgment about how much time, effort, and patience they have for daily living with a child or adult with disabilities is essential for constructing a realistic physical therapy plan. Knowledge such as parental activities that foster a child's continued development, parents' financial and emotional capacities for adapting their homes to facilitate a child's mobility, or for purchasing toys that help progress a child's development is vital for constructing valid physical therapy assessments. Unrealistic or unachievable goals help no one. In fact, they often result in a parent's decision to discontinue physical therapy or resistant behaviors, from both parent and child, none of which helps the child.

In a word, parents are invaluable for physical therapy assessment and treatment because of the reality they bring to the situation. Therapists, on the other hand, need to be adept at distinguishing honest, trivial, and unrealistic responses of parents. Physical therapists, like all team members, need to be sophisticated in communication techniques, emotional support techniques, and setting goals that are likely to be achieved when parents and therapists work harmoniously for the same child's benefit.

Physical therapists cannot accurately or thoroughly evaluate a child's consistent performance of self-help activities such as bathing, feeding, dressing, walking, and equipment usage without a parent's honest assessment of the child's daily performance of those activities in the home environment.

Physical therapists, like those who worked with Kathleen and Tommy, whose cases are discussed later, understand the value of mobilizing parents and professional colleagues as advocates for children's future independent living. Parents with intuitive, innovative ideas for their children's welfare need the support of physical therapists in implementing them. Environmental and equipment adaptations, physical and emotional support to discipline children to perform daily functions, and preparation for adulthood are possible with parental participation in interdisciplinary service of physical therapists.

Parents who advocate effectively for their children also provide needed pressure on physical therapists to initiate referrals to health professionals such as orthopedists and neurologists, speech pathologists and nurse practitioners. Parents, in collaboration with physical therapists and other team members, can work wonders with their children. Alone, neither parents, physical therapists, nor other colleagues can achieve goals for functional independence and possible future employment of children with disabilities.

TYPICAL PARENT QUESTIONS/COMMENTS OF PHYSICAL THERAPISTS

As a parent who happens to be a professional, I have had the "them and us" attitude frequently. I know that I started learning about disability the day my son was born but not through any college course. How can we professionals do our part not to judge and categorize parents?

This question carries us back to the history of physical therapy education and practice. This parent's lament is contemporary evidence of the continuing dominance of the objective, scientific explanation of disease and its structure of therapeutic relationships based on control by health professionals. That is, emphasis on discipline-specific diagnostic and treatment protocols acknowledges the authority of professionals but disregards the authority of the child and of the parents. When professionals express this attitude about their knowledge and skills, they are unable to honor the participation of children and families. The result is the "them and us" dichotomy that this parent described. This tradition is the foundation upon which education for most health professionals has been structured throughout the twentieth century.

The belief that health professionals are experts who have learned all they need to know about children with disabilities through academic education alone is gradually being challenged and replaced in medical and allied health education communities. Medical, nursing, and allied health education is increasingly restructured to foster attitudes of shared power, shared responsibility, and shared participation in collaborative programs. They are increasingly designed to help children and adults with disabilities develop and mature as partners in a humane society. Much credit for this shift goes to the Pew Health Professions Commissions, which have been working for over a decade to challenge traditional health care curriculum models.

The Commissions' reports recommend restructuring health professions' education to focus on individual life styles, to increase emphasis on behavioral sciences, and to recognize the value of nonprofessionals in providing health care. Those reports also recommend increased attention to life-span issues. Parents of infants and children with disabilities are acutely aware that their children will likely become adults someday. When they are adults, these former children will need to be able to live as independently as possible, especially if they survive their parents.

An encouraging outcome of the Pew Commissions Reports is development of community-campus partnerships that provide educational experiences for health professionals in communities (not in academic health sciences centers) where students become active participants in the civic and family lives of local residents. This kind of service-learning experience is one giant step toward ending the split between health professionals and families during long-term care for children with disabilities. Service-learning also fosters development of collegial relationships among health professionals, children, and families. Because it is experience-based and occurs outside the classroom, service-learning is achieving attention of educators and practitioners alike.

Gradually, physical therapy educators are implementing academic and clinical experiences for physical therapy students that focus on collaboration. With increased time in clinical education, service-learning, and community-based experiences throughout the curriculum, physical therapy students have more opportunities to acknowledge, understand and value the feelings and contributions of parents and children they serve. This evolving model breaks the barrier between "them" and "us." It makes all of us partners in the project of improving quality of care and quality of life for children with disabilities.

_____

Dr. Schulz's Response:

This parent/professional's question reminds me of the attitudinal difference I found after I had gone back to college and had become a professional. I was the same parent who was concerned about the same child and yet I was treated with far more respect than I had been in the past. I am glad that a focus on collaboration is evolving.

_____

We are a very active family and participate in a wide variety of sports. I'd like to have social and recreational outlets for my child with physical disabilities. What resources are out there and how do I access them?"

Community resources for children with exceptionalities vary considerably across the nation and within counties and states. Here are some resources that should be easy to contact in most communities.

1. Public school systems often provide social and recreational programs. Contact your local school principal's office or the local parent teacher association for guidance and identification of local resources.
2. Voluntary health and human service organizations, such as Easter Seal, United Way, American Red Cross, The Salvation Army, United Cerebral Palsy, county Associations for Retarded Citizens (ARC), Boy Scouts and

Girl Scouts, and local police or firemen's organizations may sponsor recreational projects for children with disabilities. The yellow pages of your local telephone directory are probably a good place to start.

3. Some churches sponsor recreational programs, classes, and services for families and children that may provide you with social and recreational contacts for your child.

4. In many communities, local social service agencies (such as United Way or the Chamber of Commerce) provide resource books that list local agencies and services for persons with disabilities, children and youth, and senior citizens. These resource books provide valuable information for pursuing recreation and social programs in a community.

5. Parent support groups, government-sponsored city and county recreation parks, and civic groups such as Rotary and Kiwanis clubs are also good places to look.

6. Horseback riding stables sometimes provide hippotherapy, or horseback riding for children with disabilities. Check your local telephone directory for information about places that offer riding opportunities for children and adults. They might be familiar with hippotherapy and, if not, you could get them interested in starting a program using local high school students as volunteers to help ride with the children.

7. Finally, if you have access to the internet, you may find directories of services, organizations, and support groups for children with disabilities and their parents that can lead you to local resources. Following is an internet address for services in the greater Pittsburgh, Pennsylvania area that can get one started on this search. Although one might not live in the region, this web material provides many good ideas about community services and how to approach finding the right resources for a child and family. http://www.pitt.edu/~uclid.ucdhome.htm

---

Dr. Schulz's Response:

The question concerning social and recreational opportunities is a critical one. While there are many opportunities in cities for children who have disabilities, in small towns and rural areas these activities are frequently unavailable. Probably the most logical approach is through the school. In one small town, the physical education teacher has made a concerted effort to include all children with disabilities in her program. She has instituted a buddy system enabling all students to be of assistance to those who may need help in some way. The result is a program satisfying to all students. Such activities also lead to strong social ties.

The PT who works with my child is wonderful. The activities she uses, however, often look painful. Does all that movement of children's arms and legs during treatment hurt?

What looks painful isn't necessarily painful to the child. Here are some reasons why this might be the case with your child. During stretching of tight muscles, children may experience discomfort when the physical therapist works with them. The same may be true when a child has been chair-bound or inactive for other reasons. Children sometimes feel afraid to move in patterns or positions they are not used to assuming. Fear may cause them to resist physical therapy exercises or to react as if they feel pain. Excessive muscle tone, such as rigidity or spasticity, might require strenuous activity on the part of the therapist during an exercise session. Resistance to the therapist's work in this case can be traced to the muscle tone and its reflexive pulling back against stretching. Reflex resistance often appears to be a withdrawal from pain.

Ask your physical therapist to demonstrate on you so you can feel what your child's body experiences during a physical therapy session. Therapists usually work within a child's comfort level and do not exceed that level without compelling reasons. Ask the physical therapist to explain what he or she is doing and why. An explanation should help you understand what your child might feel and why the appearance of pain may be merely an appearance.

Finally, if your child has an area such as a shoulder or leg that is, in fact, sore or painful, try beginning an exercise session on an area some distance from the sore area or joint. For example, if your child's shoulder hurts, begin exercising his or her elbow or wrist and gradually move up to the shoulder during an exercise or play session. Exercising in the bathtub is also a good way to diminish pain during exercise of a joint or muscle that is sore.

CASE EXAMPLE

Tommy

Sarah was the mother of Tommy, not quite three years old. She brought him to the center for interdisciplinary evaluation and follow-up. Sarah's primary concern was improvement in Tommy's mobility around the home. During the evaluation session, Tommy had numerous temper tantrums and refused to cooperate with anyone, including his mother. A realistic picture of Tommy's motor function was impossible under these circumstances.

Sarah was a careful observer of his daily behavior and she reported honestly her perceptions of his abilities to get around in their home. Sarah, therefore, became the primary source of accurate, dependable information and judgment. Using her assessments, comments, and requests, the physical therapist was able to establish a realistic physical therapy plan for purchase of a wheelchair and walker for Tommy. Sarah stated that she and her husband were able and willing to redesign the interior of their home to accommodate the wheelchair and walker. Her husband also built a wheelchair ramp and learned to fold up Tommy's chair for transport in the family automobile when they took trips away from home.

Tommy's grandmother took care of him during weekdays while Sarah was at work. The grandmother was aging and unable to carry Tommy around the house. Teaching him to use a wheelchair and walker therefore allowed Tommy, his grandmother, and his parents to live with him without risking injury to their backs from constant lifting or carrying him from room to room. For Tommy, his wheelchair and walker meant that he could independently move about the house, join his family in activities away from home, and take part in the life of his community.

In this situation, the mother's honest and accurate reporting of her son's functional abilities made possible the achievement of a goal (Tommy's independent mobility using a wheelchair and walker) that would not have been considered by the physical therapist if her evaluation information had been confined to observation of Tommy' s disruptive behavior during one evaluation session. Furthermore, Tommy's enhanced mobility at home allowed the occupational therapist and a special educator to work with his mother and grandmother to improve his feeding and constructive play activities. This latter point also demonstrates how physical therapy intervention enhanced Tommy's ability to participate in other activities recommended by members of the interdisciplinary team.

Kathleen

Parents typically play additional roles in optimal interdisciplinary service of physical therapists. Kathleen's mother played those roles beautifully. Kathleen was eight years old at the time of her first interdisciplinary team evaluation. She was able to walk without assistance but had poor balance and endurance. She fed and dressed herself most days but sometimes she wanted her mother to dress and feed her, and to stay at home with her instead of insisting that Kathleen attend classes at the daycare center.

Kathleen's mother wanted the physical therapist and other team members to make Kathleen take care of herself and go to class every day. After a congenial and thorough evaluation of Kathleen's motor ability to perform consistently and continuously her daily functional activities, the physical therapist met with team members and Kathleen's mother. They discussed the need for Kathleen's mother to reinforce daily that Kathleen was able to prepare herself for daily classes at the day care center.

In this case, reinforcing Kathleen's ability to independently groom herself and walk was preparation for her adulthood. Kathleen's ability to daily

attend classes at age eight was essential for her later participation in employment and independent living arrangements. Those abilities needed to be
reinforced daily by Kathleen's mother to build confidence, discipline, and
self-advocacy for Kathleen. Having determined that Kathleen had the motor
ability to take care of her daily functional needs, the physical therapist was
able to enlist the support of team members and Kathleen's mother in a program of daily reinforcement of functional independence. At the same time,
the physical therapist and other team members served as authority figures,
relieving Kathleen's mother of the total responsibility for insisting that
Kathleen prepare herself at eight years old for productive life as an adult.
Furthermore, the physical therapist and team members were able to support
and strengthen Kathleen's mother in her preparation of Kathleen for further
self-reliance.

Stories like Kathleen's and Tommy's illustrate the varied roles that parents
play in optimal interdisciplinary practice of physical therapy. In both cases,
the physical therapist determined the children's functional abilities with the
help of their mothers. Following physical therapy evaluations, the therapist
was able to share her findings with team members so they could all work
together for the child's benefit. And those collaborations proved helpful for
Kathleen and Tommy's present and future lives.

This next case, based on a real child and family, further emphasizes the
importance of early intervention and physical therapy programming to
improve a child's functional abilities and preparation for adult living.

Sheila

Sheila was five years old when she began physical therapy. She was diagnosed with cerebral palsy and mental retardation soon after birth. Sheila is
now seventeen years old. Her story emphasizes the importance of participation in community recreational activities, parental advocacy, and early physical therapy assessment and treatment consistently followed throughout a
child's school years. When Sheila was five years old, she was wearing a
straight leg brace and could move around her house and community with
assistance of a wheelchair and walker. Her mother became a strong advocate
for Sheila and other children in the community who needed special services
while they attended the local school. Thanks to her mother's tireless efforts,
Sheila was able to have physical therapy at school each of her twelve years
as a student in the local public school.

Sheila's mother also advocated throughout the community for development of recreational programs for children with disabilities. As a result of
those efforts, Sheila and her friends were able to participate in special

Olympics programs, to swim in the pool at the local YMCA, to go horseback riding while attending summer camps sponsored by the local Association for Retarded Citizens (ARC), and to compete in races for children in wheelchairs.

Because she became physically and socially mobile in her community, Sheila was able to enroll in vocational training programs sponsored by a local organization. At age fifteen, she moved from her mother's home to a group home where she has lived the past two years. She is now employed full time in a local industry and commutes to and from her group home using wheelchair-adapted transportation services sponsored by the local ARC. Sheila now earns a salary and lives away from her family home in an environment adapted for her disability, her employment abilities, and her future growth as an adult.

Without her mother's strong advocacy in the community, Sheila could have been confined to a more dependent future, to a lifetime of limits instead of relative independence and assumption of adult responsibilities.

There were times during her early years in physical therapy, especially after surgeries on her leg and foot, that Sheila did not want to participate in her physical therapy exercises and activities. She complained of pain during her exercises and was reluctant to try new activities for fear they, too, would hurt. But her mother's persistence and the sensitivity of the physical therapist and other team members helped Sheila continue her physical therapy program. Her mother's persistence also was responsible for Sheila's regular attendance at the physical therapy clinic, for her participation in follow-up services at school and at home, and development of community recreational and social services for children with disabilities.

Sheila's physical therapist also persisted. She was sensitive to Sheila's fears and often adapted treatment sessions to foster Sheila's trust and participation in her own exercises. The physical therapist's sensitivity to Sheila's emotional and social needs sometimes meant that physical therapy sessions included more play and less exercise, more talking and less action, or more attention to her mother than to Sheila.

Sheila, her mother, and the physical therapist, by working together and with others on the interdisciplinary team, were able to help Sheila grow to young adulthood with promise for her relative independence as an adult.

Acknowledgment

Gratitude is expressed to Marion Reinsch, physical therapist, for her valuable assistance in preparation of clinical materials, insights and experiences that helped ground this chapter's content in current practice with children with developmental disabilities and their families.

Editors' Note:

White points out an exciting trend in preprofessional training for physical thera-pists. Specifically, she notes the recommendations of the Pew Commission which sup-ports movement from traditional training to education emphasizing service-learning. We concur with White's assertion that service-learning is a valuable step toward pre-service preparation that will foster professional-family collaboration.

REFERENCES

Grover, K. (Ed.). (1989). *Fitness in American culture: Images of health, sport. and the body, 1830-1940.* Amherst, MA: The University of Massachusetts Press and Rochester, The Margaret Woodbury Strong Museum.

Murphy, W. (1995). *Healing the generations: A history of physical therapy and the American Physical Therapy Association.* Alexandria, VA: American Physical Therapy Association.

Nagi, S. (1991). Disability concepts revisited: Implications for prevention. In A. Pope & A. Tarlov (Eds.), *Disability in America: Toward a national agenda for prevention* (pp. 309-327). Washington, DC: National Academy Press.

O'Neil, E. H. (1993). *Health professions education for the future: Schools in service to the nation.* San Francisco: Pew Health Professions Commission.

Pew Health Professions Commission. (1995). *Critical challenges: Revitalizing the health professions for the twenty-first century.* San Francisco: UCSF Center for the Health Professions.

Shugars, D. A., O'Neil, E. H., & Bader, J. D. (Eds.). (1991). *Healthy America: Practitioners for 2005 an agenda for action for U.S. health professional schools.* Durham, N.C.: The Pew Health Professions Commission.

World Health Organization. (1980). *International classification of impairments, disabili-ties, and handicaps.* Geneva: Author.

Chapter 8

AUDIOLOGY

SANDY KEENER

It is estimated that over 20 million Americans have some degree of hearing loss. Included in this estimate are at least 8 million school-age children who are hard of hearing or deaf (Berg, 1986). In fact, 1 in every 1,000 infants born has profound hearing loss, with even more frequent occurrences of lesser degrees of hearing loss (American Speech-Language-Hearing Association, 1993a).

There are three basic types of hearing loss. A conductive loss is one that results from problems with the outer and middle ear. The loss fluctuates due to poor sound conduction. The most typical type of conductive hearing loss results from fluid collection in the middle ear. This is typically addressed through medications or surgery. In contrast, a sensorineural hearing loss is caused by problems with the inner ear or less frequently the nerve pathways to the brain. The loss is permanent and results in faulty sound perception. That is, the outer and middle areas of the ear conduct sound appropriately but the damaged inner ear does not send a clear acoustic signal to be perceived by the brain. The final type of hearing loss is of mixed origins and shares conductive and sensorineural characteristics.

Regardless of the type of hearing impairment, hearing loss occurs on a continuum. Typically, degrees of loss are described using the terms slight, mild, moderate, severe, or profound. These terms refer to the loudness levels and pitches heard by persons with hearing loss. Obviously, the greater the loudness level required for hearing and the greater the restrictions on pitches heard, the greater the degree of loss reported. Loudness levels and pitches are charted on an audiogram by an audiologists. Loudness is charted in decibels and pitch is charted in frequency.

MAJOR ROLES AND RESPONSIBILITIES OF AUDIOLOGISTS

Audiology is the study of hearing; audiologists are the professionals trained in the field of audiology. Audiologists have a strong background in communication sciences and disorders. They are trained regarding the normal sequence of communication and auditory development and what may enhance or inhibit normal development. Audiologists may specialize in a specific area of the field such as prevention, diagnostic evaluation, amplification and rehabilitative services, as well as educational, industrial, or recreational audiology. Audiologists may also have expertise with a particular population such as pediatrics or geriatrics. They may be involved in a variety of duties including audiometric testing, fitting and dispensing hearing aids, providing rehabilitative services and administrative duties. Common places of employment include private or public hospitals, schools, rehabilitation facilities, private practices, or in the offices of an ear, nose, and throat physician. Prevention, identification, assessment, and rehabilitation are discussed below as typical roles of the audiologist.

Prevention programs are established to conserve the normal function of the auditory system and to educate people on how to safeguard against preventable hearing loss. Audiologists dealing in prevention may, for example, develop and implement services to conserve hearing of infants in neonatal intensive care units. They may also go to industrial sites to work with employers and employees on programs to help guard against hearing loss caused from overexposure to intense noise during work.

Identification programs focus on screening various populations in order to target individuals with, or at risk for hearing loss. Early identification of hearing loss is vital and leads to the need for effective identification programs to be established. The National Institute of Health (NIH) (1993) recommends that all infants be screened for hearing loss within the first three months of life. The NIH recommends this universal screening because the use of high-risk factors as a screening tool identifies only half of newborn hearing loss. Despite this recommendation, lack of personnel and financial constraints dictate that many facilities only screen infants who show risk factors for hearing loss. Early identification programs take place in neonatal intensive care units and newborn nurseries. Screening programs are also a part of public schools, health departments, government agencies, and industry. Hearing loss may develop at any time during a person's life. In addition to screening services, identification programs provide information regarding various topics in order to help educate people about hearing and hearing loss.

Although prevention and identification programs are vital, many audiologists focus on the assessment and rehabilitation of hearing loss. Accurate and early diagnosis of hearing loss is critical in order to minimize its impact on communication in academic, social, and vocational functions. Young children and children with developmental disabilities are often difficult populations to accurately test and thus may not be served by all audiologists. This is due, in part, to limitations in audiology clinical set-up, as well as audiologists' lack of experience with these populations. An accurate and reliable assessment of hearing often requires more than one audiologist, expensive and technical equipment, and knowledge of developmental disabilities. Depending on the severity of the disability and the level of participation from the client, tests and procedures will vary.

Regardless of the tests used to evaluate hearing, the diagnostic session should begin with a case history. Case history information is typically provided by parents and review of any available medical and school records. This history helps the audiologist determine which test procedures may be most helpful and best to start with. For example, if parents report that their child has had ear problems and dislikes having his or her ears examined, the audiologist should be prompted not to begin with a physical examination of the ears or any other tests that involve immediately touching the child's ear. Although these tests are necessary, they may be easier to obtain and be less invasive once rapport has been established and the child feels more comfortable.

The assessment procedures chosen will vary depending on each individual child. The success of behavioral hearing tests is dependent on the cognitive and functional level of the child. Behavioral Observation Audiometry (BOA) is a subjective measure of auditory function, typically used for infants, which utilizes noise makers to elicit a behavioral response such as a startle. This procedure is not widely used because it is not considered an accurate measurement of hearing ability and generally fails to identify those with less than severe to profound hearing loss. For infants, children functioning at less than the five- to six-month level, and children whose behavior prevents accurate subjective assessment, the Auditory Brainstem Response (ABR) and Otoacoustic Emissions (OAE) are considered reliable and objective measures of auditory function.

The ABR is obtained under natural sleep or, if necessary, sedation. Rapid clicks are delivered to each ear, separately, at varying loudness levels. The brain's response to these clicks is measured. The softest stimuli to elicit a response is called the threshold, which correlates with hearing in the high pitches. The ABR does have limitations: it is generally expensive, it typically reflects hearing in the high pitches only, it cannot determine type of hearing loss, and it does not tell us if the child understands sounds.

The measurement of OAEs gives information about the function of the hair cells in the inner ear and the correlation with hearing. It is also most successful when the child is asleep or sedated. The presence of emissions suggests normal hearing or borderline to minimal hearing loss. The absence of emissions suggests at least a mild hearing loss. The limitation of OAE testing is that it cannot, by itself, pinpoint the amount or type of hearing loss. It can, however, give information about low, mid and high pitches.

For children functioning from six months to two years, behavioral audiometric testing can typically be done in the sound booth, using speakers (or earphones if the child will allow). A typical procedure used is called Visual Reinforcement Audiometry (VRA) and uses operant conditioning and reinforcement of a response with a visual stimulus. A variety of sounds and speech can be used. Some limitations are that the testing usually requires two examiners, one in the room keeping the child's attention and the other operating the equipment. Unless the procedure is done using earphones, ear-specific information is lacking.

The most complete information about hearing can typically be obtained using earphones for children who function at the two-year level or above. This testing involves some type of conditioned response to a variety of sounds. A comprehensive assessment includes measurement of speech threshold, pure tone testing, word recognition testing, and middle ear function.

The rehabilitative services provided by an audiologist are as important as the accurate assessment of a child's hearing. Rehabilitative services have two main components, amplification and programming. These components involve many steps that vary, depending on the age and developmental abilities of the child.

The first step in treatment of hearing loss is a referral to an otolaryngologist (ear, nose and throat physician) for a complete assessment to determine cause of hearing loss, if possible, and if medical or surgical treatment will improve hearing. In cases when medical treatment is not warranted, the physician signs a medical clearance for the child to be fitted for amplification.

If a family chooses amplification for their child, the audiologist will provide the selection, fitting, and dispensing of amplification and other necessary assistive devices. Hearing aid selection is based on many factors, including type and degree of hearing loss, as well as physical aspects and behavioral considerations. Sometimes physical deformities prevent optimal placement of a hearing aid. Some children do not tolerate placement of a hearing aid in their ears. In many cases, a team approach is necessary to assist families in financial, social and behavioral aspects of hearing aid usage. At the time of fitting, an orientation is provided to teach parents proper use and care of the hearing aids. The orientation may also involve a daycare provider, educator, or other persons involved with the child.

As soon as hearing loss is identified and decisions are being made for amplification, the second component in treatment, referral for programming, is initiated. Programming for persons with hearing impairment involves techniques to develop and/or improve communication skills. These are generally referred to as aural rehabilitation/habilitation programs. Although the audiologist has significant input regarding programming considerations, other disciplines are essential in assisting the family to plan an appropriate program. There are no straightforward guidelines to follow when selecting an appropriate program. Many considerations must be taken into account when choosing a program, particularly for children with other delays unrelated to hearing loss. Decisions are made to determine whether or not intervention will include sign language in addition to spoken language. This approach is referred to as total communication and combines the use of hearing with visual presentation of language. Another educational approach is referred to as auditory-oral in which emphasis is placed entirely on the auditory system to develop speech and language. Still another approach relies solely on manual communication. The decision regarding the best approach is an issue of much controversy. Despite the choice, children who are hard of hearing or deaf, for whom amplification is chosen, should be encouraged to use their residual hearing maximally.

CONTRIBUTIONS OF AUDIOLOGY TO INTERDISCIPLINARY PRACTICE

Hearing loss may have a negative impact on language development, speech production, and speech perception. Deficits in these areas may, in turn, negatively impact on cognitive development, social skills, academic performance, vocational choices, and family relations. Recent figures suggest the prevalence of hearing loss in children from birth to 18 years of age is 5 percent (American Speech-Language Hearing Association, 1993b). Many children with hearing loss have additional sensory impairments, neurological problems, and developmental delays. Some reports have suggested that approximately one-third of persons with hearing loss have an additional handicapping condition (Cherow, Diggs, & Williams, 1982). Based on these figures, auditory services are often essential for children with developmental disabilities. The audiologist is needed to educate other team members, families, paraprofessionals, and others about the risk factors for congenital and acquired hearing loss, behavioral indications of hearing loss, and the need for assessment. They are also essential in providing consultation to classroom teachers and vocational counselors.

Audiologists have comprehensive knowledge of normal auditory function, hearing loss, associated difficulties, and appropriate intervention. The role of the audiologist, as a team member, is to determine the type and amount of hearing loss, estimate how much the hearing loss is contributing to developmental delays or behavior concerns, determine need for habilitation or rehabilitation, and make recommendations for medical follow-up. The audiologist works closely with parents and other professionals or agencies to ensure that a child's hearing ability is maximized. Through a comprehensive interdisciplinary team approach, the audiologist is provided information about global development and medical issues that may impact decisions regarding appropriate assessment and intervention recommendations. In turn, the audiologist can provide other team members, who rely on an accurate assessment of auditory status, important sensory information to assist them in making their diagnostic impressions.

For example, if a child has a hearing loss, this will significantly impact his or her ability to perform tasks with auditory instruction. In addition, a child's ability to attend to tasks will be significantly compromised. A hearing loss must be ruled out as the cause of poor performance on auditory items on an IQ test. A speech-language pathologist relies on an accurate hearing assessment to make impressions regarding speech and language delays. Before assuming that all difficulty on a motor evaluation is due to delay, the physical and occupational therapists must be assured that their verbal instructions weren't compromised by a hearing loss. A referral for behavior management may be considered in a different light if a significant hearing loss could help explain why a child was impulsive, had a short attention span or did not respond to parent commands.

The audiologist also works closely with other disciplines and family members in determining intervention needs. For children under the age of three, infant/toddler programs are common and emphasize parent-infant training. These programs may be center-based or home-based. The philosophy behind these programs is that parents are their child's natural teachers, and learning takes place in a natural environment. This type of programming utilizes activities to increase auditory awareness and teaches that there is meaning attached to sound. The audiologist's role is to clearly communicate the child's auditory abilities and needs to the parent/infant team for their consideration.

Children age three to five are typically referred to preschool programs. Again, programming is determined with input from the referring team members who collaborate with the educational audiologist, speech-language pathologist, hearing-impaired consultant and special educator regarding programming options. Emphasis is placed on activities that will encourage expressive language, concept development, social skills, and preacademic readiness. Many preschool programs have students both with and without hearing. Some preschool programs are noncategorical where children with a variety of disabilities are served.

Educational placement for school-age children varies but may include residential schools for the deaf, private schools or public schools. Mainstreaming students with hearing loss as a primary disability is becoming more common due, in part, to Individual with Disabilities Education Act (IDEA). Consultative services are provided by the educational audiologist, speech-language pathologist, and/or teacher of children with hearing impairment.

THE ROLES PARENTS TYPICALLY PLAY IN THE OPTIMAL INTERDISCIPLINARY SERVICE PROVISION OF AUDIOLOGY

Hearing loss is often not apparent at birth. Most children who are hard of hearing or deaf are born to hearing parents. Approximately half of children with hearing impairments have no apparent risk factors that lead one to look for a hearing loss. Hearing loss cannot be identified on a routine medical exam; it must be specifically evaluated. Parents are often the first to suspect that their child may have a hearing loss. They provide essential information to the audiologist about their child's responsiveness or lack of responsiveness to sound.

Parents are an essential component of the assessment process as well. During the hearing assessment, a parent is typically in the sound booth with the child either in the lap or close by in a chair. Parents can help comfort their children in a room that often appears scary to children. They can provide information as to whether the child's participation in the activity is typical. During word recognition testing, they can help by informing the audiologist whether or not a picture or word presented to their child is familiar. In clinics where there is not a second audiologist, the parent is taught that role. Parents can assist in the evaluation by giving their child blocks and turning pages in a test book. The audiologist, then, is in an adjoining equipment room, helping the parent through the process via headset worn by the parent.

If a young child is identified as having a hearing loss, the parent's role is a significant one. A medical examination of the child must be obtained to rule out any medically treatable conditions that could be causing the hearing loss. This can lead to multiple appointments with an ear specialist. If the hearing loss is not medically treatable (the majority of sensorineural losses are not) the parents may choose to have their child fitted with hearing aids. Parents assume the majority of duties related to hearing aids. They are typically the ones putting hearing aids in and taking them out. They are responsible for keeping them in working order, checking that they are functioning and most of all, keeping them on their child. In many cases, the parents are financially responsible for the hearing aids, which can cost from $800 to over $2,000 per aid.

It is widely agreed that parents are their child's natural teachers and that parental involvement in children's programming is essential. Parents of children who are deaf or hard of hearing are faced with making a decision about what type of communication they want their child to use and be taught. A child can be placed in a totally oral program where auditory input is exclusive. A child may be placed in a totally manual program where language is taught through signing. A parent may choose a total communication program where the child is taught speech and language through whatever modality is most effective for the child. In many cases, the parents must learn a new communication system such as sign language.

Professionals and parents must work closely together to ensure that parents understand their child's hearing loss. The audiological evaluation is filled with technical terms and technical equipment. It is the audiologists' responsibility to accurately convey the information to the parents using lay terms and written materials or pictures when needed. It is the parents' responsibility to ask for clarification when it is not understood. Both parties have important information to bring to the evaluation and treatment of the child and must educate each other in their area of expertise.

TYPICAL PARENT QUESTIONS/COMMENTS FOR AUDIOLOGY

My child has autism. I've heard several things about Auditory Integration Therapy (AIT), and I don't know what to believe. What can you share about this and its potential value for persons with autism?

Auditory Integration Therapy (AIT) is considered a controversial listening treatment/therapy for hearing inconsistencies. As opposed to a standard treatment, a controversial treatment is not based on sound scientific research or data that support its claims of effectiveness. AIT is based on the work of a French otolaryngologist, named Guy Berard, and has only recently been introduced in the United States. It was initially used for children with autism, but now some advocates of the procedure claim benefit in treating other problems including central auditory processing disorders, attention deficit hyperactivity disorder, and learning disabilities, to name a few (Berard, 1993).

The original theory behind AIT is that extreme auditory sensitivity interferes with cognitive processing abilities and that this extreme sensitivity can be documented by testing a child's hearing. According to Berard, the audiograms of some children with disabilities show "peaks and valleys" of 5 dB to 10 dB difference in adjacent frequencies, thereby indicating the child hears certain pitches better than others. This, in turn, causes auditory distortions AIT claims to eliminate. To document a change, the audiogram is repeated midway and at the end of therapy. According to Berard, the midway audiogram allows for any necessary adjustments in filters based on changes in the audiogram. During AIT the child listens to music which is filtered and modulated to not give sound to "hypersensitive" areas and to exercise other areas according to the audiogram. AIT consists of the child listening to a total of ten hours of electronically modulated music presented through earphones over a ten-day period. There are typically two half-hour listening sessions per day with several hours in between sessions (Berard, 1993). The cost of AIT is approximately $1,000.

This theory, as well as the use of AIT, has been challenged for many reasons. It is generally agreed that there is no evidence to support that a peripheral auditory abnormality is an underlying condition in autism. Also, obtaining a reliable audiogram on a child with autism is very difficult. A study of 199 subjects failed to obtain a reliable audiogram on 55 percent of the subjects (Rimland & Edelson, 1994). In addition, a plus or minus 5 dB variation in threshold is accepted as a normal variation whereas larger variations are commonly seen in populations that are considered difficult to test. The current AIT devices deliver amplified sound to listeners whose hearing sensitivity is often unknown. This could be problematic in that measurements are not taken to determine the loudness of the sound in the listener's ear to ensure it is safe.

Although many professionals challenge AIT, others support it. Some advocates of AIT suggest that changes in listening behavior are seen because AIT uses more central processing energy than normal listening. Therefore, it reorganizes the processing system to allow more energy for listening and attending after treatment (Lucker, 1997). Edelson and Waddell (1991) conducted a study with 17 children and adolescents with autism. They reported positive changes in auditory memory, attention span, comprehension, impulsiveness, distractibility, echolalia, and self-stimulating behaviors. They did not report a change in the audiograms of the participants. Supporters agree that more scientific studies are needed in the area of AIT and indicate that these studies are currently taking place.

Monville and Nelson (1994) surveyed parents whose children had received AIT. Of the surveys sent out, 27 percent were returned. Of the small group who did respond, 50 percent reported a positive change in behavior control and 70 percent reported a positive change in reduction of sound sensitivity problems. Fifteen percent of the parents reported a negative change in behavior control.

The lack of scientific data to support AIT contributes to the controversy surrounding its claims. However, professionals are obligated to inform parents about all treatment options, whether or not they endorse them.

An audiologist evaluated my daughter with mental retardation at age two. Although the results suggested she could hear, this first contact with a member of the professional community started a series of other evaluations leading to her eventual diagnosis. It is my suspicion that the audiologist had a good idea what the diagnosis would be, but was reluctant to share it with me until other parties became involved. Why do you think she was reluctant?

As a part of their educational training, audiologists take extensive coursework relating to development, particularly in the area of auditory and communication skills. Because they have been trained on age-appropriate development and behaviors, as well as deficits in these areas, they recognize when possible delays are apparent.

As previously noted, subjective tests administered by an audiologist require specific developmental skills in order for valid and reliable results to be obtained. For example, children with problem-solving abilities at age two to two and a half typically can be conditioned to respond to auditory signals under earphones. They should have communication skills that enable them to participate in basic speech recognition testing. When an audiologist tests a child and must significantly alter age-appropriate tests due to developmental limitations of the child, concern regarding the child's developmental status should be noted. Despite their knowledge of development, the audiologist should take care not to draw conclusions based on limited experience with a child. Children may not give their best performance for many reasons other than developmental delay. They may be frightened by the test booth, may be fearful of the earphones used in testing or may be uncooperative during the procedure. The audiologist should discuss his or her observations and concerns with parents and make recommendations for evaluation when appropriate.

When parents seek audiological services, it is often due to concern over communication development, in addition to lack of consistent response to sound and speech. When a hearing loss is ruled out as a possible cause for these concerns, other explanations must be sought. The responsibility of the audiologist is to assess hearing status and make appropriate referrals to other disciplines when developmental delays are suspected. An audiologist cannot assess cognitive, motor, or communication development or make diagnostic statements about those skills. They can and should, however, convey their concerns regarding these other aspects of development when they are noted.

I've been to several professionals in pursuit of care for my child. The question I have relates to why they don't communicate better with each other. I don't know how many times I've been asked to convey the same information. Do you have any suggestions for your peers as to how we can eliminate some of this redundancy?

This is a common complaint from parents whose children are seen by many professionals. When individual service providers evaluate children, these concerns are more apparent because providers are typically in different physical locations. Reports from one service provider may not reach the next service provider before the child is seen. Additionally, professionals may not be accustomed to working together and sharing information in this type of arrangement.

The advantage of many interdisciplinary teams is that all service providers work together in the same physical location. The interdisciplinary process of evaluating a child should help alleviate some of the redundancy parents face when telling their story. When interdisciplinary assessments are scheduled, complete records for that child should be obtained well in advance of appointment dates. The professionals involved in the assessment of the child should review these records. In some settings, a case coordinator is assigned to review the records and complete a written summary for others. The individuals scheduled to see the child would have this summary and review the child's chart. Despite this preparation, the professional should have the parents expand, clarify and update information, if necessary. Because children evaluated in an interdisciplinary setting are seen by multiple professionals individually, parents and children may still be left to tell the same thing over and over. Good communication between the members of an interdisciplinary team should help in this regard.

When children are seen in an "arena" assessment, many professionals are in the same room with the child being tested and are there together to hear the parents answer questions. They may gain their assessment information by observing a child being tested by a related professional. For example, young children receiving developmental testing often receive an arena assessment where a psychologist, speech-language pathologist, and occupational or physical therapist work together to evaluate a child. This type of assessment is not, however, appropriate for all evaluations. The use of an arena assessment is typically dictated by the age and developmental/behavioral abilities of the child.

Professionals should advise parents to keep detailed records on their children. They should have information and reports from any assessment their child has released to them and keep these organized in a notebook. A professional involved in assessment of a child being seen by multiple service providers should be aware that parents are being asked redundant information and that this information is sensitive and often difficult to constantly retell.

Dr. Schulz's Response:

The author's suggestion that parents keep a notebook is excellent. We all kept records when our children were babies: notations about their weight, feeding, inoculations and other important events. When you discover your child has a disability, this practice should be continued. It doesn't need to be lengthy, just timely and accurate. This notebook, then, can be shared with each professional, who can make a copy if necessary. To facilitate team work, professionals could add comments to the notebook.

CASE EXAMPLE

AJ is a two-year, three-month-old female referred for an interdisciplinary team evaluation by her pediatrician due to parental concerns regarding speech and language delays and hearing ability. Due to the family's concern about AJ's hearing, the audiologist on the team was chosen as evaluation coordinator for this case.

The case history was completed from a review of the medical records sent from the pediatrician, birth records from a local hospital, and a family interview. This information was compiled and presented by the evaluation coordinator. A preassessment staff meeting was conducted with members of the interdisciplinary team to provide input as necessary.

AJ lives at home with her parents. She has a three-month-old brother. Her mother is a homemaker and her father is a sales manager for a large company. The family has private insurance that covered the planned assessment.

AJ was the product of a full-term, uncomplicated pregnancy and vaginal delivery. She was discharged as a healthy newborn after a 24-hour hospital stay. Neonatal health history was unremarkable. According to the high-risk register completed prior to AJ's discharge from the nursery, no factors associated with hearing loss were identified. The hospital did not have a universal screening program. AJ was followed medically for well-baby visits and her immunizations were up to date. Medical history was significant for recurrent otitis media and one upper respiratory infection, which were treated with antibiotics.

Developmental milestones were reportedly normal for motor development. However, delays were indicated in the areas of communication and auditory development. At age 27 months, AJ was reported to have less than a 50-word vocabulary. She communicated primarily through gestures and her speech was difficult to understand.

Behaviorally, AJ was described as having a limited attention span and was difficult to discipline. Her parents were questioning whether her slow speech and language development and ignoring behaviors were due to the "terrible twos" stage. In order to address the physicians and the parents concerns, professionals from the following disciplines were asked to evaluate AJ over a two-day assessment period: developmental medicine, audiology, speech-language pathology, and psychology.

AJ was found to be a healthy child. Her physical growth was within normal limits. Her neurological exam was normal. Some unusual physical features were noted but were not felt to be significant. Her ear exam revealed normal physical appearance of the eardrums.

The hearing test was performed under earphones; however, Visual Reinforcement Audiometry was used because AJ could not be conditioned to respond reliably by dropping blocks. The hearing exam showed responses to speech at 20 dB HL in the right ear and 25 dB HL in the left ear. These responses are considered in the borderline normal to slight range of hearing loss. Responses to tones were in the borderline to slight hearing loss range in the low pitches. Beginning at 2000 Hz, a moderate sloping to severe hearing loss was measured in both ears. Testing was attempted using the bone oscillator in order to identify the type of hearing loss; however, AJ would not tolerate placement of this headset. AJ's responses to speech were reflective of her better hearing in the low pitches and testing was considered reliable. Word recognition testing was not performed due to reported limited vocabulary. Tympanograms were obtained to evaluate eardrum mobility and were normal in both ears. Although the type of hearing loss cannot be determined without measurement of bone conduction thresholds, the normal tympanograms and normal medical examination, which preceded the hearing test, would make a conductive hearing loss unlikely. The hearing test was the second assessment completed on AJ. The findings were conveyed to the speech-language pathologist and the psychologist prior to their appointments with AJ.

A battery of standardized tests for vocabulary comprehension, expressive language abilities, and speech production assessed communication abilities. Informal observation and structured play were also used. The speech and language assessment revealed significant speech and language delays characterized by reduced language comprehension and limited expressive language abilities. Multiple articulation errors were noted which were felt to coincide with the frequencies for which hearing loss was noted.

Psychological assessment revealed low average performance on nonverbal measures of intelligence. Verbal IQ scores were significantly lower and were commensurate with the findings of speech-language pathology. A limited attention span was noted particularly during verbal measures and instruction. AJ could be redirected easily with gestural prompts accompanying verbal prompts. The psychologist reported that the results should be interpreted with caution due to the reported hearing loss, as the performance on nonverbal items required verbal instruction.

The above findings were discussed in a post assessment staffing with input from all disciplines involved and AJ's parents. Based on the information provided by the interdisciplinary assessment and input from the family, the following recommendations were made.

AJ was referred to an ear, nose and throat (ENT) physician by her primary care doctor. The ENT was requested to medically evaluate a possible cause of the hearing loss, rule out medical treatment and provide medical clearance for hearing aids. In addition, recommendations for genetic counseling were made to assist in diagnosis of the cause of the hearing loss due to lack of high risk factors.

Following the ENT exam, AJ was scheduled to return for ongoing audiological testing to attempt to obtain responses using the bone oscillator. In addition, hearing aid selection was pursued, which required multiple visits for hearing aid fitting, orientation, and follow-up. Behind-the-ear hearing aids were selected, which allow flexibility. According to the family, their insurance covered the cost of hearing aids.

Referral was made to a parent-infant program, which offered a center-based program for children who are hard of hearing. The program emphasized a total communication approach, which the team and parents felt would be appropriate for AJ. She attended this program three mornings per week. The program was staffed by a teacher who was hearing-impaired, a speech-language pathologist and an early childhood special education teacher. A home visit took place for one hour, one time per week. In addition, a parent group met one time per week for one hour (during the center-based instruction time) to discuss issues the parents have identified as important to them.

Follow-up speech-language and cognitive assessments were recommended for six months following hearing aid fitting and programming. Audiological testing of AJ's three-month-old brother was recommended as no high-risk factors were noted in AJ's history and a hearing loss should be ruled out in her sibling.

Editors' Note:

Keener does a nice job of describing the importance of hearing to overall development. Most of us fail to realize the interrelatedness of hearing impairment to other communication, cognitive and social deficits. In sum, it is imperative that parents and professionals alike, look for signs of hearing loss in children with suspected delays. Given that the procedures of the audiologist are reliable and relatively simple, early assessment can go a long way toward clarifying effective interventions for children with and without hearing loss.

REFERENCES

American Speech-Language Hearing Association. (1993). Guidelines for audiology services in the schools. *ASHA, 35*(10), 24-32.

Berard, G. (1982). *Hearing equals behavior.* France: Masionneuve.

Berg, F. S. (1986). Characteristics of the target population. In F. S. Berg, J. C. Blair, J. H. Viehweg, & Wilson-Vlotman (Eds.), *Educational audiology for the hard Of hearing child.* New York: Grune & Stratton.

Cherow, E., Diggs, C., & Williams, P., (1982). Demographics and description of the problems. In E. Holzhauer, K. Hoff, & E. Cherow (Eds.), *Hearing impaired and developmentally disabled children and adolescents: An interdisciplinary look at a special population* (pp. 11-122). Rockville, MD: American Speech-Language Hearing Association.

Edelson, S. M., & Waddell, L. L. (1991). Auditory training and the auditory training project. Unpublished manuscript. (Available from S. Edelson, Ph.D., Director, Center for the Study of Autism, 2207 B. Portland Rd., Newberg, OR 97132).

Lucker, J., & Miller, M. (1997). Auditory Integration Training. *American Journal of Audiology, 6,* 25-32.

Monville, D., & Nelson, N. W. (1994). Parental Viewpoints on Change Following Auditory Integration Training for Autism. *American Journal of Speech Language Pathology, 3*(2), 41-54.

National Institutes of Health (1993). Consensus Statement. Washington, D.C. Rimland, B., & Edelson, S. M. (1994). The Effects of Auditory Integration Training on Autism. *American Journal of Speech-Language Pathology, 3*(2) 16-24.

Chapter 9

SPEECH-LANGUAGE PATHOLOGY

DEBORA BURNS DANIELS

Speech-language pathologists provide diagnostic and intervention services to individuals with communication disorders across the life span. Speech-language pathologists identify, assess, diagnose, and treat speech, voice, language, communication, and swallowing disorders (American Speech Language Hearing Association (ASHA), 1996). Professional requirements include a master's or doctoral degree and the Certificate of Clinical Competence (CCC-SLP) from ASHA. In addition to obtaining a graduate degree in speech-language pathology, professionals must pass the National Examination in Speech-Language Pathology and Audiology and successfully complete a Clinical Fellowship Year. Speech-language pathologists and clinical fellows who are members of ASHA must follow ASHA's Code of Ethics. This code defines professional responsibilities for the provision of highest quality services to all consumers (ASHA, 1996).

In addition to achieving the Certificate of Clinical Competence, speech-language pathologists in 46 states must also meet requirements for state licensure. Furthermore, speech-language pathologists who work in public school settings may be required to meet additional state requirements for teacher certification. The credentials CCC-SLP (Certificate of Clinical Competence Speech Language Pathology) signal to the consumer that the professional has met the requirements designated by ASHA as necessary for the provision of quality services.

MAJOR ROLES AND RESPONSIBILITIES OF THE SPEECH-LANGUAGE PATHOLOGIST

Speech-language pathologists have multiple responsibilities, including the prevention, identification, assessment, diagnosis, and treatment of communication disorders. Professionals also counsel patients and family members about communication deficits and work collaboratively with other therapists to develop effective diagnostic and intervention programs. In addition, speech-language pathologists serve as clinical instructors and supervisors in university settings, and/or participate in research in the area of communication disorders. Speech-language pathologists are employed in a variety of settings such as hospitals, university clinics, private agencies, public schools, home health agencies, and public health departments. ASHA notes that over 50 percent of speech-language pathologists work in school settings, while another 39 percent are employed in health care facilities, and 4 percent work in university or college settings (ASHA, 1997).

Speech and language therapy services to infants, toddlers, and school-age children have expanded over the past twenty years. The original and reauthorized Individuals with Disabilities Education Act (IDEA) has greatly increased the number of children who receive special services, such as occupational, physical and speech-language therapy. The U.S. Education Department reported in 1995 that more than 5.4 million children were provided special services under IDEA. Approximately 21 percent of all students receiving services under IDEA had a primary diagnosis of speech or language impairments. However, 75 percent of all children served under IDEA received speech-language therapy (U.S. Department of Education, 1995). These speech-language therapy services were provided in a variety of settings, such as homes, Early Childhood Special Education preschools (ECSE), community preschools, daycare centers, public schools, hospital and university clinics, and other private agencies.

The speech-language pathologist shares the responsibility for prevention of communication disorders with other professionals such as physicians and audiologists, as well as with patients and family members. Identification of potential problems at a very early age may reduce the impact or severity of the communication disorder by beginning treatment as soon as possible. Prevention activities typically consist of public service announcements, presentations about speech-language development to parents and professionals, and printed, family-friendly materials regarding typical communication development.

Communication disorders consist of problems in one or more of the following areas: speech, language, social interaction, and feeding/swallowing. Speech disorders involve phonology and articulation (sound production and associated rules), vocal quality, and fluency (effortless speech production without pauses, hesitations, repetitions, etc.). Children with language impairments may exhibit problems with comprehension, vocabulary, and grammar. They may also have difficulty using language in context. For example, they may have limited interest or understanding of how to use their language to interact with others. Finally, the survival of medically fragile children often results in a need for modified or alternative modes of nutrition. Because of their specialized training, speech-language pathologists also are being asked now to evaluate the safety of a child's feeding and swallowing, and to make recommendations for interdisciplinary management of nutrition issues.

It is often the parents or a primary caregiver who feel that something is not quite right with a child's communication or feeding skills. Speech-language pathologists employed by hospital clinics or school districts are usually available to consult with a parent by phone to determine if a potential problem exists and to suggest appropriate actions. It is helpful to have collected some key pieces of information when consulting a speech-language pathologist, such as a description of the current concern, when the problem began and how it has developed over time. It is also important to know how the communication problem interferes with social interactions and school performance (Morris, 1994). For a young child, the speech-language pathologist may also ask questions regarding other developmental skills, such as when the child began walking or was toilet trained. Parents may be confused about questions that do not seem to be related to a communication problem. Obtaining other information will help the speech-language pathologist decide whether the problem warrants immediate assessment or if some suggestions for home activities might be appropriate with professional follow-up at a later date.

The speech-language evaluation process remains the same for each type of communication problem, while the assessment tools may vary according to the specific concern. The speech-language pathologist identifies the referral concerns, collects background history, and develops an assessment plan. The actual assessments will be some combination of interview, skilled observations in structured and unstructured tasks, and administration of norm-referenced tests. Ideally, the child's performance might be observed across multiple contexts or settings, so that a clear picture of communicative abilities with a variety of partners/settings emerges. Observation across multiple settings is sometimes difficult to arrange due to time or travel constraints. However, in those cases the speech-language pathologist may ask a parent or referral source to provide videotaped samples of the child's performance. Another option might be for the speech-language pathologist to interview (in person or by telephone) caregivers, teachers, and others or ask them to complete written questionnaires in order to create a complete picture of communication skills.

Using a family-centered approach, the speech-language pathologist typically begins an assessment with a discussion about the significant people in the child's life and how the communication problem impacts his/her relationship with those significant people. A variety of reasons for the communication problem may emerge. Subsequently, the speech-language pathologist will ask for a specific description of the behavior(s). Questions about when the problem was first noted, the consistency of its presence/severity over time, and how the problem has been addressed prior to this evaluation will be included. A history about speech and language and general developmental milestones is collected. The speech-language pathologist may also ask if other family members have had communication and/or learning problems. For some specific speech and language disorders, information about general health will be necessary. The detailed history taken about health, growth, and development will suggest a specific diagnostic plan for the interdisciplinary team.

When selecting an assessment battery, the speech-language pathologist reviews the referral concerns and the information collected to date. Other factors to consider include the time and setting in which to conduct the evaluation and the examiner's ability to establish rapport with the child. With young children, evaluations may need to be conducted in familiar surroundings and completed over several sessions in order to minimize fatigue. A school speech-language pathologist may spend some time visiting in a student's classroom or chatting with the student before beginning the actual evaluation process. The use of interesting toys or conversational topics often aids the interaction between the child and speech-language pathologist.

Assessment tools include interview, informal and/or structured observational tools, norm-referenced and criterion-referenced tests. Norm-referenced tests provide information on the expected skill level of a specific population. For example, The Peabody Picture Vocabulary Test-III (Dunn & Dunn, 1997) provides information about vocabulary comprehension skills. A child's performance on this formal measure may be compared to that of other children the same chronological age if the test has been administered in the prescribed way. The speech-language pathologist compares the child's performance to same-age (and in some cases, same sex) peers. Many times, it is the child's performance on norm-referenced measures that is used to determine eligibility for special services.

The speech-language pathologist uses both norm-referenced and criterion-referenced measures. As mentioned above, norm-referenced tests compare the child's communicative performance to that of other children of the same age. A criterion-referenced tool, however, allows the speech-language pathologist to compare the child's current level of performance to previous performance, looking for specific gains in individual skills. Criterion-referenced measures provide specific, detailed information on speech-language skills that can be used for planning intervention and assessing progress.

In addition to more formal measures, the speech-language pathologist incorporates skilled observation as part of the assessment battery. Skilled observations provide information about the frequency and quality of specific communication behaviors. Those settings and communication partners who maximize the child's performance can be identified. This is valuable information when developing an intervention plan.

To summarize, the communication assessment process is individualized, based on the concerns reported by the parents or referring agency and the case history information collected. The battery will most likely be a combination of skilled observation, interview, and administration of formal test measures. Once the information is collected, the speech-language pathologist will analyze it to develop a diagnosis.

The speech-language pathologist uses a problem-solving approach to develop the assessment plan. The interpretation of the diagnostic information may yield a diagnosis for the communication problem. However, results may also lead to the need for additional measures or referrals in order to establish an accurate diagnosis. Often, impaired communication is noted to be part of a larger developmental or medical problem. The diagnosis of a speech-language delay/disorder may be secondary to medical or other developmental issues.

After a diagnosis is obtained, speech-language pathologists participate in the development of an interdisciplinary treatment plan. Speech-language pathologists provide intervention services to children and adults in a variety of settings, using multiple service delivery models. Such settings include home, hospital clinics, university clinics, private practices, school classrooms, early childhood programs, and daycare settings. Typical delivery models include direct therapy, consultative models, home-based services, center-based services, community-based services, inclusion settings, and collaborative models. There are strengths and weaknesses with each of these models. Ultimately, service delivery should be based on a commitment to serving children in the environment that best fits their individual needs (Blosser & Kratcoski, 1997). The intervention team, including the parents, speech-language pathologist, and other team members as needed, should work together to identify the components of the child's intervention program.

Traditionally, speech-language therapy services have utilized a pull-out model, where children worked with a speech-language pathologist individually or in small groups, several times per week. These services were typically conducted in an area away from the student's classroom, if provided at school, or in a small therapy room in a clinical setting. However, as special education services have moved from restricted settings into regular education classrooms, school and clinical speech-language therapy services have also changed. Regular education classrooms, home and community-based settings are now considered to be the least restrictive environment for the provision of speech-language therapy services. Once again, the intervention program should be tailored to meet the needs of the individual student. A combination of classroom and pull-out services may be appropriate for one student, while another student thrives in a totally inclusive setting.

CONTRIBUTIONS OF SPEECH-LANGUAGE PATHOLOGY TO INTERDISCIPLINARY PRACTICE

Early childhood special education programs provide services to infants and young children with a wide variety of handicapping conditions. The early childhood special education teacher, occupational therapist, or speech-language pathologist working alone could never meet all of the special needs of young children with disabilities. Peterson (1987) recommended that best practice for service delivery to infants and young children incorporates interdisciplinary and/or transdisciplinary service provision. Interdisciplinary practice involves specialists who work together in serving the same children by meeting, planning, and coordinating services (Peterson, 1987). This collaborative service model has been increasingly used with school age children as well, in order to provide education in the least restrictive setting. ASHA describes collaborative or interdisciplinary practice as the opportunity to: (a) observe and assess how the student functions communicatively and socially in the regular classroom, (b) describe the student's communicative strengths and weaknesses in varied educational contexts, and (c) identify which curricular demands enhance or interfere with the student's ability to function communicatively, linguistically, and socially (ASHA, 1991). In transdisciplinary service provision, one individual serves as the primary service provider to deal directly with the child. Peterson (1987) notes that transdisciplinary service provision continues to require interdisciplinary evaluation and program planning, but that the implementation of that plan is carried out by one team member, in consultation with other professionals. Transdisciplinary service delivery models are likely to be used in providing treatment to infants and toddlers. Very often, speech-language pathologists participate on interdisciplinary diagnostic and intervention teams, and may also serve as consultants or the primary service provider in a transdisciplinary setting.

Team members share certain responsibilities in any interdisciplinary setting. Common roles shared by team members include: (1) equally participating in team decisions about educational priorities and interventions for the child, (2) joint problem-solving across all areas of the child's program planning, (3) sharing discipline-specific knowledge to maximize the child's performance on targeted objectives and to increase team understanding of the child's abilities, (4) actively supporting the knowledge and skills of other team members, and (5) continuing to seek out additional training that would support/maximize the child's performance in all settings (Rainforth et al., 1992). In a collaborative or interdisciplinary setting, the speech-language pathologist brings specific knowledge to the team about the developmental progression of speech, language, social interaction, play, and cognitive skills. Professional training encompasses the neuromotor functions associated with oral motor skills for speech, eating, swallowing, breathing, and voicing that complements the training of the physical and occupational therapists. Finally, speech-language pathologists are able to design intervention programs for those children requiring alternative or augmentative communication (Rainforth et al., 1992).

Traditionally, speech-language pathologists have functioned in a medical model, where they received referrals from physicians, parents, teachers, and others. They tested the child and developed intervention plans specifically related to speech and language deficits. Intervention was completed in individual or in small group sessions several times a week. Current changes in health care and educational reform have encouraged movement away from a traditional therapy model to approaches that are more functional in nature. The PAC Model (Providers, Activities, and Contexts) represents a framework for choosing individualized intervention strategies (Blosser & Kratcoski, 1997). In this model, the speech-language pathologist first determines the key communication partners for the child, what roles they might play in the intervention process (e.g., model appropriate communication behavior, data collection, etc.), and what training is required in order for the communication partners to feel comfortable in those roles.

Blosser and Kratcoski (1997) note that the PAC model may be used by the speech-language pathologist to assist interdisciplinary teams in a variety of settings, including infant/toddler home-based services, preschools, schools, hospitals and clinic settings. In an interdisciplinary setting, the speech-language pathologist is often called upon to consult with other team members. Consultations may occur formally or informally. For example, the speech-language pathologist may be asked to observe a student with severe and multiple disabilities in his or her regular education classroom and to make suggestions about ways to increase appropriate opportunities to gain the attention of his or her peers. The intervention team might ask the speech-language pathologist to help prepare a social story (Gray, 1994) to assist a child with autism in making a successful transition from the classroom to the lunchroom. The Headstart preschool teacher may consult the speech-language pathologist for assistance in developing a classroom social skills curriculum. An occupational therapist might request suggestions from the speech-language pathologist for maximizing communication opportunities during range of motion activities for a child with cerebral palsy.

Occasionally parents are concerned that their child with special needs is not receiving enough individual speech-language therapy. It is important to recognize that communication opportunities occur 24 hours a day, making it impossible for the speech-language pathologist to be present at all times. Thus, as an interdisciplinary team member, it is the responsibility of the speech-language pathologist to develop a treatment plan that can be implemented across environments and communicative partners. To make the implementation of that plan successful, the speech-language pathologist must provide adequate information about how the individual's communication problem impacts or may be impacted by different persons/settings to other members of the interdisciplinary team. The speech-language pathologist should model these intervention techniques for other team members. Finally, the speech-language pathologist must be available to observe and provide feedback to other team members carrying out the communication intervention program with the child. The responsibilities described above are at least as or more important than the actual provision of direct services by the speech-language pathologist.

THE ROLES PARENTS TYPICALLY PLAY IN OPTIMAL INTERDISCIPLINARY SERVICE PROVISION OF SPEECH-LANGUAGE PATHOLOGY

Paget (1992) states that, "The importance of family-school partnerships to the quality of a very young child's early education cannot be overstated" (p. 119). This premise also applies to the relationships between families and individual therapists such as the speech-language pathologist.

Typically, it is recommended that professionals encourage families to express their own thoughts about how the child's communication problem is impacting the family, what goals they have for their child and what type(s) of intervention strategies seem most workable at home. Professionals are encouraged to be proactive and knowledgeable about the family cultural background, offering culturally sensitive forms of help instead of waiting for families to ask for assistance. Team members are encouraged to include family members at all levels of the decision-making process, viewing the family as equal partners. Offering to schedule meeting times around parent work schedules, providing family-friendly written information about the program, encouraging frequent visitation and actual participation in treatment are additional responsibilities of the teams (Paget, 1992).

A list of parent responsibilities for team participation might be developed using the above list of professional responsibilities. First, it is important that family members openly communicate their thoughts and feelings with other team members. When teams establish a positive atmosphere, family members will feel more comfortable expressing their feelings without fear of criticism. Second, families must not assume that each team member is aware of and/or clearly understands any cultural issues that might impact the family's ability or willingness to participate in the team process. Although it is the responsibility of the professional to be culturally sensitive, families must help team members understand how those issues should be addressed. When faced with difficult decisions about other family members, or ourselves, it is often easy to want to leave the decision-making process to the professionals. Many times, families feel that they don't have the technical expertise to make suggestions about the intervention plan but later privately voice concern that not enough emphasis was given to helping their child learn to read, complete math homework, speak clearly, or meet other individual needs. Family members must share these concerns as part of the team process. Professionals and families occasionally disagree on what is the best method of intervention for a particular skill. They come to a team agreement about what is best for the child after open discussion that is respectful of the knowledge that each team member brings to the process. Parents are very knowledgeable about their children. If parents choose not to participate in the decision-making process, it is easy to become removed from active participation in the treatment plan.

Parents are often encouraged to view themselves as equal partners in the intervention program. It is important to recognize that not all parents wish to be therapists. Parents may choose not to provide direct services to their child. Yet they may still be equal partners in this process by several means. They keep themselves informed about the nature of the communication problem and the types of strategies being used. They remain equal partners, too, by carefully observing and reporting to therapists the rate at which the child is learning new skills or developing abilities. Family members must also understand that being a direct service provider does not necessarily mean sitting at a small table conducting therapy. For example, it may mean recognizing that the speech-language pathologist has been working on the development of a simple action word vocabulary, and has asked parents and siblings to emphasize those words throughout daily routines.

Finally, family members should share information with the team about how the child is performing at home. Notebooks may be sent back and forth from home to school, so that daily or weekly communication is maintained. Family members may wish to observe their child at school. It is often helpful to other members of the team to actually see how a child performs in settings other than therapy or school. Thus, families may choose to videotape their child at home, or invite team members to observe their child at home, at daycare or in other settings.

TYPICAL PARENT QUESTIONS/COMMENTS FOR
SPEECH-LANGUAGE PATHOLOGY

How do you think professionals would approach their jobs differently if it was their child who was receiving services?

Having worked as a speech-language pathologist for many years, I felt that I was skillful in working with parents, conducting family-centered assessments and developing functional intervention goals. I allowed ample time for parents to ask questions, often giving them my home telephone number, in case they couldn't reach me during the day. However, I never clearly felt the grief and frustration experienced by these families until my youngest son was diagnosed with Attention Deficit Hyperactivity Disorder in the fourth grade. As parents, we were aware that our child had problems completing work as early as first grade. We worked carefully with each teacher to put a behavior management plan in place to encourage him to complete assignments and stay on task. Our school principal helped us to choose teachers whose classrooms were very structured and predictable, and who welcomed parent participation. Our son was described in various terms as bright, loving, a comedian, immature, distractible, ornery, and "all boy." However, by the beginning of fourth grade, we could see that he was having increasing difficulty with the completion of work. We kept in close contact with his teacher by weekly phone calls and daily notes. After some initial success, things deteriorated once again. We felt frustrated that our teamwork was not having the desired result. I had been reviewing literature about ADHD and wondered if that might be a possible diagnosis for our son. This diagnosis was confirmed after an extensive evaluation by a developmental pediatrician and a behavioral psychologist.

Once the diagnosis was in place, a combined approach of counseling, behavioral intervention and medication quickly produced positive results both at home and at school. The remainder of the school year went smoothly. However, my husband and I received a variety of comments from other family members, most of which were negative (e.g., "Oh, he's just the baby," "You just spoil him too much," "Mom, you didn't let me get away with that when I was his age!," or "He doesn't need medicine, he just needs a good spanking"). We were forced to take on the role of advocates, educating other family members about ADHD, and how it impacted our son and our family. Advocacy for our son at school became our next responsibility. To be on the other side of the conference table as a parent, and not as a service provider, was a very uncomfortable feeling. I experienced embarrassment and fear that others had judged my parenting skills and found them lacking.

For the remainder of his elementary school career, our intervention plan worked smoothly. We felt confident that our son would be able to handle the transition to junior high school. However, this was not the case. Instead of handling the expectations of one teacher and one classroom, our son needed to manage the assignments/responsibilities given by six different teachers with six different sets of expectations. It wasn't long before my husband and I were receiving daily phone calls at work. Once again, intervention meetings were arranged. This time, teachers, counselors, and administrators seriously outnumbered us. Several of these individuals were neighbors or professional acquaintances. It was obvious that some faculty members were willing to work with us, while others simply viewed our son as "impulsive" and a behavior problem. From that point on, it was very clear that we would need to continue to be active educational advocates throughout the remainder of his school career. Being an educational advocate results in feelings of satisfaction when things are going well, and exhaustion, frustration, and anger when problems arise. Knowing that we will be long-term educational advocates can be overwhelming.

While it is unreasonable to suggest that all speech-language pathologists have their own child with special needs, it is possible for them to listen to families share their stories about dealing with physicians, teachers, therapists, or people from state agencies. The child with special needs is impacted in a host of ways depending on the environmental context. The child with special needs also impacts those people in his/her environment. The recognition that children both impact and are impacted by their special needs yields professionals who are supportive and flexible, rather than rigid and judgmental. Professionals who recognize the number of roles parents play (caregiver, advocate, therapist, employee and spouse) can approach families in a manner that values parent input and that facilitates respect and trust. It is ultimately trust and respect that will result in the development of a successful interdisciplinary team.

Why wasn't my child's speech-language pathologist more definitive about a prognosis regarding the probability that he would or would not eventually speak? He was first evaluated at 15 months of age, and not knowing what to expect created anxiety for our family.

The acquisition of verbal communication is related to the child's cognitive, motor and social development. Impaired hearing acuity may impact verbal communication as well. The range of what is considered to be normal or typical language development at 15 months of age is quite variable. For example, using published norms a typically developing 15-month-old female child could understand as few as 60 words or as many as 255 words and say as few as 5 words or as many as 67 words (MacArthur, 1993). For a male child of the same age, comprehension of 60 to 219 words and use of 3 to 33 words would be within normal limits (MacArthur, 1993). This variation in what is considered as acceptable performance is present across all areas of development. Parents recognize that children typically are walking at one year of age, yet there is an acceptable range of variation for learning to walk. Children do not gain skills evenly across all areas of development. One 15-month-old child might have a vocabulary of 50 words but has only been walking for about six weeks. Another child may have walked at 9 months but only says 10 words at 15 months of age. Both children display skills within the acceptable range of typical development but present different profiles. It is very difficult to provide parents with a long-term prognosis for the acquisition of verbal communication at 15 months of age, unless there are clearly recognizable factors present that are known to ultimately result in lack of or limited speech. It is important to rule out hearing loss as a contributing factor. It is more likely that the speech-language pathologist and other members of the interdisciplinary team will need to observe the child over an extended period of time, monitoring the rate of progress.

Parents are understandably worried about whether their child will develop verbal communication. Information about other areas of development, hearing acuity and health status are important factors in determining the prognosis for speech development. Rate of developmental progress over time will also impact prognosis. The speech-language pathologist will be looking at several factors to predict acquisition of expressive language skills. Initially, the severity of the deficits must be documented. The current rate and type of vocalizations can be recorded. That is, how often does the child try to communicate with other people in his or her environment, either nonverbally or vocally? Does the child frequently point to preferred items, show the father interesting toys, or reach toward objects and then look to her grandmother to direct attention? When pointing does not work does he or she add vocalizations to the requests? What types of sounds does the child currently make? Does his or her sound repertoire consist only of vowels, or are there some developmentally appropriate consonants observed? When the child does make sounds, does it appear to be effortful to move his or her tongue, lips, and jaw? In addition to those diagnostic questions, the speech-language pathologist must be aware of the condition of the child's muscle tone and whether or not it is adequate to support speech production. Finally, the speech-language pathologist must determine the child's interest in social interaction, and his or her motor and vocal imitation skills.

Information derived from answering those diagnostic questions will help the speech-language pathologist form an initial hypothesis about whether or not the child will be a verbal communicator. The information used to form this hypothesis should be shared with the family at the time of the initial diagnosis, so that they understand how such a prediction is made. It is also very important that parents understand that communication does not solely occur by speaking. The speech-language pathologist should identify the variety of ways that their child may be communicating nonverbally. The speech-language pathologist should also help parents to understand that while the ultimate goal may be verbal communication, there are many intermediate steps that will allow their child to communicate successfully. Adults must acknowledge and respond to those alternate forms of communication if their child is to have continued interest in interactions with others.

Once again, clear communication among all members of the interdisciplinary team (including parents) is essential when attempting to identify the child's current modes of communication. In addition, of those currently used, which communication modes are considered to be most socially appropriate (e.g., it is more socially acceptable to point to a desired toy than to whine or reach in the general vicinity of the toy box)? A description of the child's communicative performance across contexts should be shared with the team, so that members are consistent with their expectations. In addition, this discussion may identify which activities and materials promote increased sound production and gestural communication, so that these will be incorporated into all daily routines as is possible. The child's performance over time should be carefully documented so that team members may communicate this information to family members. Keeping family members informed helps to alleviate the anxiety about their child's communication, by clearly documenting his or her progress and giving them concrete, functional intervention strategies to use in all daily routines.

When I watch my child's speech therapy, it just looks like the speech-language pathologist is playing with her. What is going on that I'm missing?

Linder (1993) notes that, "... play is systematically related to areas of learning and development ..." (p. 24). Linder goes on to say that play and learning are interdependent, with play leading to advanced cognitive skills, which, in turn, lead to more skillful play. During play, children learn social understanding by taking the perspective of others. That is, the child can take the role of the father while playing house one day and become the next door neighbor or a mailman on another occasion. As children become skillful in using objects, actions, and feelings in complex pretend play activities, an associated increase in the complexity of language is also noted.

Speech-language pathologists provide therapy to young children in a variety of treatment models. One model utilizes play as a vehicle to promote communication and early learning. Linder (1993) reports that children with language delays are less likely to use pretend play schemes and are more likely to play by themselves, and to have reduced social interaction with peers. Because socialization, cognition, and language development are intertwined with the addition of more sophisticated play, it is essential that play skills be included as part of a program plan for the young child with language delay.

CASE EXAMPLE

The M family's 18-month-old daughter, Jenny, was not talking. Their pediatrician referred them to the local Infant-Toddler Services Program for developmental assessment. What could they expect from this evaluation? The M's were wondering how someone can assess the communication skills of a toddler who was not talking.

Jenny's parents relocated because of Mrs. M.'s promotion at work. At their first appointment with Jenny's new pediatrician, they voiced their concerns about her lack of speech. Mr. and Mrs. M. wondered why Jenny's communication skills were so delayed. Mrs. M. felt that Jenny's chronic ear infections may have caused a language delay. Jenny's father felt that she was not getting enough individual attention at her daycare center. Jenny's maternal grandmother thought that her daughter's early return to work was the reason for Jenny's lack of speech. Jenny's pediatrician carefully reviewed her medical history and observed delays in other developmental milestones. In addition, he noted her slow rate of physical growth throughout her infancy. Although Mrs. M. had a healthy, full-term pregnancy, Jenny was small for gestational age. She had difficulty nursing, and her mother supplemented breast-feeding with formula by bottle in order for Jenny to gain weight. After multiple ear infections, Jenny was referred to an otolaryngologist (ENT) at one year of age. As part of that examination, she was noted to have a mild, bilateral conductive hearing loss by the audiologist. Jenny's ENT recommended that she have ventilation tubes placed. Subsequently, Jenny had only one ear infection in the next six months. Her hearing was rechecked six weeks after surgery and noted to be within normal limits. Jenny's new pediatrician reviewed his concerns about Jenny's growth and developmental delays and encouraged her parents to contact the Infant-Toddler Services Program.

Prior to the scheduled evaluation, the speech-language pathologist conducted a lengthy telephone interview with Mrs. M. to discuss her concerns about Jenny's communication. The speech-language pathologist also explained the evaluation process, which would consist of an arena assessment conducted by a developmental psychologist, physical therapist and speech-language pathologist. It also included an examination by the developmental pediatrician and the audiologist. The speech-language pathologist reassured Mrs. M. that she and her husband would be able to remain with Jenny during testing. Mrs. M. was asked to complete several written questionnaires ahead of time, including the Communication and Symbolic Behavior Scales Caregiver Questionnaire (Wetherby & Prizant, 1993) and the MacArthur Communicative Development Index: Words and Gestures (MacArthur, 1993). Completion of these two questionnaires provided written documentation about the quality of Jenny's communication skills, as well as a norm-referenced quantitative measure of her language comprehension and expression.

During the evaluation, Mr. and Mrs. M. remained with Jenny. The developmental psychologist conducted a transdisciplinary play-based assessment. During the assessment, the speech-language pathologist recorded skilled observations about the frequency and quality of Jenny's communication skills. These observations would be included with the information gained from the parent report forms. At the conclusion of the formal testing, the speech-language pathologist also was able to observe Jenny while playing with her parents. In addition, she had the opportunity to interview Mr. and Mrs. M. using a norm-referenced interview tool. The sum total of this information indicated that Jenny was functioning at approximately the 12-month level of development, denoting significant speech and language delays. It appeared that her profile was relatively flat, with similar delays in both language comprehension and expression. Other information gained during this assessment indicated that Jenny's motor and cognitive skills were also clustering at the 12-month level of development. Thus, while Jenny demonstrated a significant communication delay, her performance was consistent with her overall level of ability. The audiologist reported that Jenny had normal hearing, using Visual Reinforcement Audiometry. The developmental pediatrician noted that Jenny had some slightly atypical facial features, low motor tone, and poor growth. Thus, the diagnosis of speech-language delay was secondary to an overall diagnosis of global developmental delay.

Test results were conveyed to Jenny 's parents in a conference immediately after testing was completed. They were provided with hand written notes, to be followed by a formal report at a later date. Her parents were encouraged to ask team members questions about the findings. Mr. and Mrs. M. acknowledged that they had been concerned that Jenny's delayed speech was part of a bigger problem with her development. Although there was some sadness, her parents were eager to pursue medical and developmental recommendations.

Because Jenny was demonstrating global developmental delays, it was determined that she needed a comprehensive intervention plan to include speech-language therapy, early childhood special education services, and occupational therapy services. Mr. and Mrs. M. were concerned about how to arrange all of these services since both parents were working full time outside of the home. The Family Service Coordinator suggested two options. The first was to arrange for in-home therapy where the various therapists would work with Jenny and her parents in the evenings. The second option suggested was to arrange for in-home therapies at the home of Jenny's daycare provider. Mr. and Mrs. M. liked the idea of Jenny having therapy during the day, when she was most alert. They also liked the idea of including Jenny's daycare provider as a member of the intervention team. However, this arrangement did not include them as active participants in Jenny's intervention program. Mrs. M. was particularly concerned about working with Jenny on her language development. Thus, a third option was discussed. Jenny's team determined that she would receive her therapies in the home of the daycare provider. In addition, the speech-language pathologist would meet two evenings a month with Jenny's parents and grandparents to model intervention strategies.

Jenny's intervention team used the PAC Model (Providers, Activities, and Contexts) described earlier in this chapter (Blosser & Kratcoski, 1997) to develop a treatment plan. Using this model, Jenny's speech-language pathologist determined the key communication partners for Jenny, and what role they might play in the intervention process. Key communication partners included her parents, her daycare provider, and her grandparents. In addition, Jenny would also be working with the early childhood special education teacher and an occupational therapist. The speech-language pathologist identified possible roles that each partner might play (e.g., model appropriate communication behavior, data collection, etc.) and what training was required in order for the communication partners to feel comfortable in those roles. Jenny's communication partners were all very willing to take an active role in modeling appropriate language behaviors. In addition, Mrs. M. and the ECSE teacher agreed to take on the additional role of documenting Jenny's progress in acquiring new vocabulary words. The speech-language pathologist met with Jenny's team as a group to provide basic instruction about the communication strategies.

In the next step of the PAC process, a treatment plan determining specific activities and strategies was developed. Jenny's speech-language pathologist was careful to identify what steps were necessary to prepare the communication partner to use language intervention strategies and record Jenny's progress. Several home visits were made to model the strategies for Jenny's daycare provider, parents, and grandparents. In addition, opportunities to modify the strategies were discussed and practiced until her family felt comfortable. In the final step of the PAC process, specific daily routines to incorporate language intervention strategies were chosen by the speech-language pathologist with input from the remainder of the interdisciplinary team. Jenny's parents identified three daily routines where they would implement the language strategies, including the evening mealtime, bath time, and during all diaper changes. Mrs. M. indicated that, although dressing and breakfast times would be rich with language opportunities, she felt that it would be too stressful to implement those strategies during the work week. Mr. M. offered to use those strategies with Jenny on weekend mornings. Jenny's grandparents volunteered to implement therapeutic activities during their weekend visits with Jenny, specifically choosing to look at developmentally appropriate books for vocabulary enrichment. Jenny's daycare provider, ECSE teacher and occupational therapist worked together to select several developmentally appropriate play activities for her. The speech-language pathologist demonstrated how to incorporate language objectives during play times.

Jenny's intervention team was excited about the number of opportunities available each day to work on communication objectives using the PAC model. The interdisciplinary team incorporated Jenny's cognitive, self-care, motor, and play objectives into this same format. Mr. and Mrs. M. were appreciative of the team effort. Mr. M. noted that he enjoyed being part of a team but also felt more confident knowing that other team members were also responsible for implementing Jenny's communication intervention plan.

Dr. Schulz's Response:

Our acceptance of Billy's overall delay was a growth process. At first we thought, "If he could just walk, we know he would be O.K." Then, "If he could just talk ..." We hired a speech therapist who ultimately told us that his lack of language development was part of a total process. It's much easier to believe that there is a single solution, but important to know that there is not.

We need to acknowledge the importance of siblings in the development of speech and language. Billy's younger sister became his chief model and teacher as her development matched and surpassed his. Their meals together, their playing, and even their disagreements provided rich opportunities for language development.

One interesting event occurred in our family. We found that some of Billy's words and expressions were useful. For example, rainbrella seemed much more expressive than umbrella and tirvedit far more emphatic than I'm really tired of it. We refer to it as "speaking Billy."

The speech-language pathologist plays an integral role in the interdisciplinary team process. Opportunities to facilitate speech, language, socialization, and feeding skills occur in all activities of daily living. In addition to providing direct intervention services, the speech-language pathologist serves as a consultant to the interdisciplinary team by examining environmental contexts and determining the speech/language/oral motor requirements necessary for the child to be a successful communicator/feeder. Once those prerequisites are identified, direct or indirect intervention strategies may be incorporated to assist the child with successful communication. It is the role of the speech-language pathologist to educate other team members, including family, to carry out communication intervention strategies throughout daily routines.

Editors' Note:

Speech and language disorders impact every area of exceptionality. Information in this chapter will be relevant to parents and professionals in each of the other disciplines.

Because speech and language pathologists cannot be expected to become experts in every area of exceptionality, this may be an area in which the parents become teachers, furnishing information to the professional when it is sought.

REFERENCES

American Speech-Language-Hearing Association. (1997). *Highlights and trends: ASHA membership and affiliation counts for mid-year 1997.* (On-line), www.asha.org.

American Speech-Language-Hearing Association. (1996). Scope of practice in speech-language pathology. *ASHA, 38* (2), 16-20.

American Speech-Language-Hearing Association, Committee on Language Learning Disorders. (1991). A model for collaborative service delivery for students with language-learning disorders in the public schools. *American Speech-Language-Hearing Association, 3* (33), (Suppl.).

Blosser, J., & Kratcoski, A. (1997). PACs: A framework for determining appropriate service delivery options. *Language, Speech & Hearing Services in Schools, 28*, pp. 99-107.

Dunn, L., & Dunn, L. (1997). *The Peabody Picture Vocabulary Test, Third Edition.* Circle Pines, MN: American Guidance Service.

Gray, C. (1994). *The new social story book.* Arlington, TX: Future Horizons, Inc.

Hohman, M., Banet, B., & Weikert, D. (1979). *Young children in action.* Ypsilanti, MI: The High/Scope Press.

Linder, T. (1993). *Transdisciplinary play-based assessment.* Baltimore: Paul H. Brookes.

MacArthur. (1993). *The MacArthur Communicative Development Inventory: Words and Gestures.* San Diego: Singular.

Paget, K. (1992). Proactive family-school partnership in early intervention. In Fine, M. & Carlson, C. (Eds.), *Family-school intervention: A systems perspective.* Boston: Allyn & Bacon.

Peterson, N. (1987). *Early intervention for handicapped and at-risk children.* Denver: Love.

Rainforth, B., Fork, J. & MacDonald, C. (1992). Foundations of collaborative teamwork. In Rainforth, Fork, & Macdonald (Eds.), *Collaborative teams.* Paul H. Brookes.

U.S. Department of Education. (1995). *Who is served by IDEA-Diverse students with diverse needs.* Testimony of Richard W. Riley, Secretary, U.S. Department of Education, to the Subcommittee on Early Childhood, Youth and Families.

Wetherby, A., & Prizant, B. (1993). *The Communication and Symbolic Behavior Scales Caregiver Questionnaire.* NJ: Riverside.

Chapter 10

ASSISTIVE TECHNOLOGY

BETH DALTON MOFFITT

Assistive technology (AT) is any piece of equipment or product system that is used to increase, maintain, or improve functional abilities of individuals with disabilities (Technology and Related Assistance Act, 1988). Assistive technology allows children to participate more fully in their school, community and society by improving their communication, their ability to complete activities of daily living and their control of environments. Assistive technology may involve an adaptation of an existing piece of equipment or a person's environment or requiring an entirely separate piece of equipment which is new to the child and his or her family.

Assistive technology is a broad umbrella term that includes thousands of devices used for many purposes. Some assistive technology solutions are considered "low tech," such as a cardboard communication board or a rubber pencil adaptation. Other solutions are considered "high-tech," such as voice-output computer communication systems or infrared environmental control systems. Assistive technology is constantly changing. Some of the low-tech assistive technologies have successfully helped many individuals for several years. The high-tech assistive technologies seem to grow and change frequently each year. It takes commitment by assistive technology professionals to stay abreast of changes.

When used correctly, assistive technology can be very helpful to the child and his or her family. Whatever assistive technology solution is selected, it should make the child's life, and subsequently his or her family's life, easier. Assistive technology should be designed to assist the child in living life to his or her full potential.

One term that is included within assistive technology is augmentative and alternative communication (AAC). Augmentative and alternative communication is frequently discussed in this chapter. It is defined as "an area of clinical practice that attempts to compensate (either temporarily or permanently) for the impairment and disability patterns of individuals with severe expressive communication disorders" (ASHA, 1989).

MAJOR RESPONSIBILITIES AND ROLES OF ASSISTIVE TECHNOLOGY SPECIALISTS

The major responsibility of assistive technology specialists is to prescribe and support assistive technology solutions. This occurs in conjunction with the assistive technology evaluation, which is defined by federal law as a functional evaluation in the potential user's customary environment (Technology and Related Assistance Act, 1988). Functional evaluations consist of obtaining information regarding motor, cognitive, language, and sensory skills and describing the person's environments. Information may be obtained from recorded reviews, interviews and/or evaluations of potential assistive technology candidates. For children, a description of environments provides information specific to the child's activities and assistive technology solutions for those activities.

The assistive technology specialist has the responsibility of coordinating training for the child, family, and staff regarding the use of assistive technology. This training may be provided by the specialist or arranged for via assistive technology manufacturers or other professionals. Regardless of where the training occurs, the fact that it occurs is imperative. The best fit assistive technology solution may be unsuccessful unless appropriate training is completed.

Finally, the assistive technology specialist is responsible for following the child and family after implementation of the assistive technology solution. By conducting follow-up, the assistive technology specialist will be able to assist with problem-solving if the assistive technology solution is not meeting the child's needs. This follow-up also allows the assistive technology specialists to actually see their prescription of assistive technology in action.

CONTRIBUTIONS OF ASSISTIVE TECHNOLOGY SPECIALISTS TO INTERDISCIPLINARY PRACTICE

Ideally, assistive technology is fit by an interdisciplinary team. Teams can consist of a variety of professionals, such as a speech-language pathologist, an occupational and/or physical therapist, a regular and/or special education teacher, a social worker, a physician, a nurse, a psychologist, an audiologist as well as others. Consultation with additional professionals may occur as needed.

The type of assistive technology evaluation, in part, determines which professionals participate. For example, an evaluation to determine the best way to access the computer for a child with left hemiparesis (weakness) with normal cognitive and language skills may only involve an occupational therapist. However, an evaluation to determine equipment needs for a preschool age child with cerebral palsey targeted for inclusion, may involve several professionals.

The location of the evaluation site may also determine the professionals on the assistive technology evaluation team. For example, a team at a school may consist of a speech-language pathologist, an occupational therapist, a physical therapist, a regular and/or special education teacher, a psychologist, and a paraprofessional. In contrast, an assistive technology evaluation team at a rehabilitation hospital may have a smaller core team consisting of a speech-language pathologist and an occupational therapist. This core group would be able to consult with a variety of professionals such as a physical therapist, a physician, a nurse, a psychologist, and/or an audiologist, as needed.

There is no consistency across evaluation sites regarding the number and type of professionals on the assistive technology evaluation team. Any professional may develop a passion for assistive technology. Also, on many assistive technology evaluation teams, there is overlap between the roles of the specific professionals on the team. For example, during an augmentative/alternative communication assistive technology evaluation, the role of the typical occupational therapist would be to determine the best way for the child to access the augmentative/alternative communication device. However, if the occupational therapist had completed several assistive technology evaluations, he or she may also be asked to describe the function of different devices. Likewise, the speech-language pathologist may be observing the child's body position while using the device. This cross-discipline assistive technology evaluation assists with meeting the needs of assistive technology users.

THE ROLES PARENTS TYPICALLY PLAY IN THE OPTIMAL INTERDISCIPLINARY SERVICE PROVISION OF ASSISTIVE TECHNOLOGY

Parents play an integral and equal role both in the assistive technology evaluation and the selection of the assistive technology solutions. Parents certainly know their child best. They can describe the need for the assistive technology and convey their child's hopes, values, likes, dislikes, background, capabilities, interests, environments, communication needs, and other needs. Parents can assist with problem-solving specific to determining which assistive technology solution is best if more than one is available.

Blackstone (1992) suggests that parents come, if possible, with stated objectives for the assistive technology. For example, the following items would be objectives for an augmentative communication device:

- must provide an efficient way to engage in conversational exchanges;
- must have the ability to create, store and retrieve messages, produce written work, and access computers; and
- must permit keyboard access, using index finger on left hand (Blackstone, 1992).

By contributing this information during the assistive technology evaluation, parents can be helpful in selecting the most appropriate assistive technology solution.

Parents are also consumers in the assistive technology process. They first gather information in order to select an appropriate assistive technology evaluation site. During the evaluation, parents must be active participants in the discussion and selection of the assistive technology solution, given their eventual responsibilities specific to the implementation of the assistive technology. The more involved parents are in the process, the more likely an appropriate assistive technology solution will be selected and the more likely they will be happy with that solution.

In one augmentative communication evaluation, parents indicated that they were most interested in a device with a voice that sounded human. During the discussion of the different devices available to their child, they were most interested in ones with digitized speech. This information was very helpful to the evaluators. It helped them eliminate the devices with synthesized speech early in the selection process.

In another example, parents reported that their child wanted to use his hand in some manner to access the computer. The assistive technology team assessed the child's ability to access the computer with his hand, his head, and other body parts with a variety of adaptations. Because the child and the family were the most interested in the use of his hand and the assistive technology team felt that this was a reasonable access point, the team was able to adapt a switch allowing for hand access.

TYPICAL PARENT QUESTIONS/COMMENTS FOR ASSISTIVE TECHNOLOGY

I'd like to convey to professionals that they don't always act like we are all on the same side. I often feel resentment if I question what has been said or conduct research into possibilities not mentioned by the professional community. What can be done about this?

It is unfortunate that any parent would ever feel this way. Here are a few suggestions that may assist parents if they find themselves in this awkward situation.

First, it is good to remember that everyone on the team, parents and professionals alike, are on the same side. At times, if there is disagreement on the team, it may not seem that this is so. All persons are there because they want to support the child. Particularly in the field of assistive technology, professionals are there because of their passion to meet the child's needs. Sometimes, a step back to realize that everyone is on the same side can be very helpful for both parents and professionals.

How parents question a professional or propose other assistive technology options from research can make or break interactions. For example, regarding a recommended communication device, parents may be much more successful asking a question like, "What do you think of its maintenance record?" versus, "I've heard that it breaks down all the time. Why would you recommend that defective device?" Obviously, this is an extreme example, but it illustrates the difference word choices can make.

It is always good to anticipate problems in team meetings. If parents think there is going to be conflict, particularly with only one of the professionals on the team, it may be helpful to set up an appointment with this professional in advance. Ask for his or her input regarding the issue involved, then, present views in a calm and rational manner. Discussion with this professional in a one-on-one situation may be much more successful than with an audience of other professionals.

The art of compromise can also be helpful in these situations. Parents may state their point of view and a particular professional may state his or her point of view. There may be room in the middle. Again, both parties are on the same team.

Sometimes it may be helpful for parents to realize the type and number of responsibilities each professional has and the environment in which they work. Although these factors should not have an impact on any team discussion, reality suggests that the opposite is so. This is not to say that parents should necessarily become involved in the responsibilities or politics of the school or hospital. Knowledge in these areas, however, may be helpful. For example, this author has always been an advocate for students. In one position, however, there was an unusually large and unreasonable caseload. Many parents requested individual therapy sessions for their children. In some instances, this author agreed with them but was unable to provide services due to the directions received from the program director. Although parents were probably frustrated, there was nothing that could be done to meet their needs.

It may be helpful to discuss team communication strategies with other parents. One parent may be able to share a particular strategy that was not successful for him or her. By parents sharing ideas, they may find that a particular professional communicates in the same manner with all parents. Parents may also find that there might be a personality conflict with one professional.

Finally, if parents feel that they have always questioned a particular professional in a calm and rational manner, scheduled appointments to discuss more intense topics in a one-on-one situation, followed tips from other parents and compromised, and still have not resolved a particular issue to their satisfaction, then it is time to talk with the professional's supervisor. It is important, however, that parents first try to resolve conflict more directly.

Dr. Schulz's Response:

Reference to the importance of word choices and inflection used by parents is also applicable to professionals. Sometimes parents have done a great deal of research on assistive technology devices and have become quite knowledgeable in this area. Sometimes, too, they have had experiences that contribute to their frustration. Until the parents and professionals have learned to know each other, both must tread softly to ensure communication and a good relationship.

This is good advice for parents and professionals. It's a matter of respect for the other person's opinion and intelligence.

How do I know that the technology evaluation my child is to receive will be the best it can be? Are there specific things that I should look for in the qualifications of the evaluators or in their practices?

Currently, a competency certificate for an assistive technology provider (ATP) or an assistive technology supplier (ATS) is available through RESNA, the Rehabilitation Engineering and Assistive Technology Society of North America (RESNA, 1997). In addition, certificates of competency in general assistive technology with specialty areas in assistive technology for young children, assistive technology for communication, and supervision of assistive technology services are available through the Research Institute for Assistive and Training Technologies (RIATT) via distance education (RIATT, 1997). There are also many universities and colleges that offer courses in some form of assistive technology, although they may not award a particular certificate in assistive technology.

Most professionals with a vast amount of experience in assistive technology do not have the specific credentials mentioned above. They will, however, have certification via their specific professional organization, such as the American Speech-Language Hearing Association (ASHA) or the American Occupational Therapy Association (AOTA). Some of these organizations have outlined specific competencies needed to meet the needs of clients requiring a variety of assistive technology solutions (ASHA, 1989).

To begin searching for an appropriate evaluation site, parents can ask for a referral from their child's physician, school, or current education/rehabilitation team (e.g., teacher, speech-language pathologist, occupational therapist, or physical therapist). Other parents may also be helpful in finding an appropriate evaluation site. Additionally, parents can contact the technology project or the alliance for technology access resource center in their state for referral (RESNA).

Parents may want to ask who is involved in the evaluation process. They may also want to know the length of time the site has been completing evaluations and the types of assistive technology evaluations they complete. It might be helpful for parents to know if evaluations occur during one appointment or across several days. Will the evaluation be conducted at one site or in several different places in the child's typical environment? Again, either approach may adequately meet the needs of a child depending on the assistive technology solution. Most importantly, parents should ask a potential evaluation site personnel about any follow-up that is conducted beyond the evaluation. It is frequently the follow-up beyond the actual evaluation that determines how successful the assistive technology solution will be for a child.

Finally, if parents require further information, they could ask the evaluation site personnel for references from other professionals or previous clients. Some sites may also allow you to observe an evaluation. Many sites, however, may not be able to give you the names of previous clients or allow you to observe due to confidentiality.

My child has a severe communication impairment and significant physical disabilities. We have obtained a good augmentative and alternative communication (AAC) evaluation for him, but now find ourselves in a maze of possible funding sources. What tips do you have for evaluating funding resources?

Ideally, evaluators should guide parents through the funding process. If the evaluators cannot help, they may be able to refer you to someone or some agency who can. Most importantly, parents need to identify a client advocate to be in charge of funding. This individual may be a parent or a professional but should be someone with a successful history of obtaining funding for assistive technology. Funding success can be 100 percent dependent upon the perseverance of the client advocate (Prentke Romich Company, 1998). If parents need additional assistance with finding a client advocate or the funding process, they can refer to the technology project or the alliance for technology access resource center in their state. Parents also may want to contact Closing the Gap, P. O. Box 68, Henderson, Minnesota

56044. Additionally, there is at least one course on funding available from the Research Institute for Assistive and Training Technologies.

Most parents will start the funding process with their school district. According to the Office of Special Education Programs (OSEP), the school district is responsible for making certain assistive technology is available and in good repair if it is part of the Individualized Education Program (IEP). The IEP team, then, needs to determine that the assistive technology is needed in order for the child to receive a "free and appropriate education." If assistive technology is needed, IEP goals should be written specifically for assistive technology. Here are a few examples of IEP goals written to include assistive technology:

- The student will self-dress using a buttoning device and a sock device.
- Using an electronic communication system, the student will produce two-word phrases while role playing.
- The student will read assigned classroom materials utilizing a scanning and screen-reading (with speech output) system (Missouri Assistive Technology Project, 1995).

With regards to funding a device parents should also remember that the school district cannot categorically deny access of assistive technology to the student according to the law. Furthermore, school districts cannot require use of health insurance if the family will incur any financial loss which includes, but is not limited to:

- an increase in premiums or the discontinuation of the policy,
- an out-of-pocket expense such as the payment of a deductible or percentage of coinsurance incurred in filing a claim, and
- a decrease in available lifetime coverage or benefit under an insurance policy (Missouri Assistive Technology Project, 1995).

On the other hand, it may be a good idea for parents to approach the school district, suggesting a funding partnership. Parents should not necessarily offer to pay for the assistive technology solutions. They may, however, be more successful with the school district by offering to be partners in securing funding for assistive technology rather than demanding that assistive technology be purchased.

Aside from, or in addition to the schools, an obvious source of assistive technology is the child's health insurance policy. Parents will need to inquire as to what information the insurance company will need to consider for payment. Many companies need the assistive technology evaluation report and an extensive description of the assistive technology solution. Letters of support from the child's physicians and therapists can also be helpful. Just as school districts may not be interested in paying for assistive technology solutions that are considered medically necessary, insurance companies are less likely to fund assistive technology solutions for educational benefits. Providing educational benefits is not covered in most insurance policies.

For many policies, the assistive technology solution will have to be considered medically necessary. Some will cover prostheses or durable medical equipment; therefore, in any given policy, some assistive technology solutions may be covered and some may not. For example, many policies will cover an electrolarynx, a device used by some persons if their larynx is removed. This device is considered a prosthesis because it replaces a missing organ. The same policy may cover wheelchairs because they are considered durable medical equipment. This policy, however, may not cover a voice-output device used for communication because the device is not considered a prosthesis or durable medical equipment.

Finally, with respect to insurance policies, there may be little precedent to having any particular assistive technology solution covered. Parents need to be prepared to appeal denial decisions. It may be necessary for parents to follow the entire claim review process.

There are still other sources of funding for assistive technology that parents may want to consider. Medicaid may cover some assistive technology solutions as they are considered durable medical equipment. It is best for parents to contact a Medicaid caseworker for assistance if they want to pursue this source for funding. For some children, aged zero to five years, who meet the requirements, many State Bureaus of Children with Special Needs will not only pay for the assistive technology evaluation but will also pay for any recommended assistive technology solutions. These bureaus usually have their own specific regulations involving assistive technology. They may have their own evaluation sites. Again, parents will need to contact the bureau if their child qualifies. For older children, State Vocational Rehabilitation agencies may pay for some assistive technology solutions. Also, *Make A Wish* organizations have bought a variety of assistive technology solutions for children who wished for them. Parents will need to contact their local organization to determine what procedures need to be followed.

Some families, for a variety of reasons, have chosen to pay for assistive technology solutions themselves. Some have taken out loans and repay them in monthly installments. Other families have received assistance from churches, professional clubs, and other organizations. Some families have received ideas from other parents as far as what funding sources may be the most beneficial to pursue in any given community.

No matter what funding source is used, parents can always consider previously owned assistive technology equipment. Sometimes this equipment can be purchased at a reduced price, even though it is still in good condition. Contacting a state's technology project or alliance for technology access resource centers may be helpful for parents in locating previously owned assistive technology equipment.

What can I do when the system tells me CAN'T every time I turn around? My child needs technology now!

There are two reasons why the system may be telling parents "can't." One reason is, of course, lack of funding. If parents have exhausted all the external resources discussed previously, then they could decide to fund the assistive technology themselves in some manner. Ultimately, the student is your child, and if you believe your child needs assistive technology, then you must be a part of the funding solution.

Second, the system may be telling parents "can't" because the student is not ready for assistive technology. Parents then need to focus on the skills needed for successful assistive technology application and assist their child in developing those skills, if possible. Professionals who work with the child should be able to identify these skills.

CASE EXAMPLE

Cody is a five-year-old boy with cerebral palsy with left hemiparesis (muscle weakness) and developmental delay. Cody has normal hearing and needs glasses for close vision. He uses a few signs, gestures, and occasionally vocalizes, but these behaviors do not meet all of his communication needs. Improvement of communication skills is one of the goals on his IEP. According to his mother, Cody needs additional ways to communicate in order to decrease his frustration and increase his acceptance with peers.

Cody walks without assistance. He can use his right index finger to accurately, but slowly, press computer keys. He only uses his left hand to hold objects in place. His teacher reports that Cody is able to reach all areas of his desk with his right hand. He is not tactilely defensive. Cody's age equivalency on the *Peabody Picture Vocabulary Test* (Dunn & Dunn, 1973) is three years, four months. His overall age equivalency on the *Brigance Diagnoistic Inventory of Early Development* (Brigance, 1991) is five years, two months. He is able to point to upper case letters upon request (five years, five months equivalent).

For an augmentative communication evaluation, Cody's private speech-language pathologist referred Cody's family to the technology project and the alliance for technology access resource center in their state. Two evaluation sites were recommended near Cody's home. One was in a children's rehabilitation center and the other was in a rehabilitation hospital, primarily for adults. Cody's parents selected the children's rehabilitation center and scheduled an appointment for an evaluation.

Based upon the assessment which targeted motor, cognitive, sensory, and contextual issues, it was determined that Cody needed an augmentative communication device which allowed for:
• direct selection, using a keyboard,
• pictures for a symbol set,
• expandable vocabulary (300-400 words plus),

• sequencing or stringing of symbols, and
• generative voice output messages.

Five augmentative communication devices were considered. Three devices were dedicated exclusively to augmentative communication and each had varying capabilities and prices. Two devices were computer-based, which also could be used for augmentative communication.

One dedicated device weighed less than the other two, making it easier for Cody to carry. All three devices used pictures on overlays, but overlays of one device needed changing more often in order to use expandable vocabulary. One device was the most expensive. Two devices were easy to program and, because they used digitized speech, the recorded voice could be matched to Cody's age and gender. One device used synthesized speech. One device was the only one of the three that used a special strategy to help Cody remember where messages were stored. Two of the devices could be rented for a trial period.

A computer-based system was also an option. Though a portable laptop, it would need to be opened whenever he wanted to use it and closed when carrying it. It also would be more expensive than the other options because a portable computer would need to be purchased.

The team recommended one of the dedicated devices for Cody. It met all the necessary criteria. In addition, it was lighter and had the special strategy to aid with remembering where messages were stored. Furthermore, Cody's speech-language pathologist had experience in implementing its use with students. His parents also liked it best of all the devices that were shown.

Because of the communication goals in Cody's IEP, the school district purchased the device.

Editors' Note:

Moffitt makes a valid point when discussing passion as a critical variable specific to the delivery of assistive technology services. All of us have personal and professional passions. Finding an assistive technology professional with a passion for what he or she does seems not only wise, but imperative, given the rocky roads to successful assistive technology solutions. In sum, a professional with a never-say-die attitude can be the intangible factor leading to assistive technology success.

Acknowledgment: Parts of the case example are reprinted with permission of the University of Kansas Medical Center Occupational Therapy Education Department.

REFERENCES

Blackstone, S. (1992). The selection process: Ideas and strategies. *Augmentative Communication News, 5,* 4-5.

Brigance, A.H. (1991). *Revised Brigance Diagnostic Inventory of Early Development.* North Billerica, MA: Curriculum Associates Inc.

Competencies for providing services in augmentative communication. (1989). *American Speech-Language-Hearing Association, 31,* 107-110.

Dunn, L.M. & Dunn, L.M. (1973). *Peabody Picture Vocabulary Test-Revised.* Circle Pines, MN: American Guidance Service.

How to obtain funding for augmentative communication devices. (1998). Prentke Romich Company, Wooster, OH.

Issues in assistive technology. (1995). Missouri Assistive Technology Project, Independence, MO.

Judge, G. (1992). *Parent guidebook to assistive technology.* Maine Department of education, Division of Special Education, Portland, ME.

Office of Special Education clarifies right to assistive technology. (1990). Office of Special Education, Washington, DC.

Ourand, P. (1991). Funding of augmentative and alternative communication: The final step of a long journey. Presentation to the annual convention of Closing the Gap, Minneapolis, MN.

Rehabilitation Engineering and Assistive Technology Society of North America. (1997). (RESNA), Suite 1540, 1700 North Moore Street, Arlington, VA 22209-1903. Research Institute for Assistive and Training Technologies (RIATT). (1977).

Technology and Related Assistance Act. (1988).

Chapter 11

EARLY CHILDHOOD SPECIAL EDUCATION

Tom Oren

The purpose of this chapter is to provide an overview of services provided to children, birth to school age, and their families; to discuss the interdependent nature of disciplines serving this population of children and their families; and to review the roles parents assume in the process of early childhood special education. In addition, responses will be provided to questions parents frequently ask about early childhood special education. Case studies will be used where appropriate to illustrate major points throughout this chapter.

Nowhere in the educational realm does there appear to be as active a philosophy of bridging the family-professional gap as there is in early childhood special education. The intent of federal laws governing the education of young children with disabilities and resultant philosophy of family-centered practices assumes equal parent-professional partnership at all levels of policy development and decision-making.

MAJOR ROLES AND RESPONSIBILITIES OF EARLY CHILDHOOD SPECIAL EDUCATORS

Early Childhood Special Education is the practice of identifying and addressing the developmental delays, disabilities, and special needs of young children and their families. Services afforded children and families in early childhood special education are mandated under federal laws (i.e., Public Law 94-142, Public Law 99-457, Public Law 101-476, Public Law 102-119, Public Law 102-57, IDEA Amendments of 1997). These laws differentiate lead agencies for providing services to children birth through two years, and three years to school age. For children three years to school age, the state and local education agencies (i.e., school districts) oversee the provision of services. For birth through two years, different state agencies (e.g., Human

Resources, Health and Welfare, Education, Rehabilitation Services, Developmental Disabilities) have been designated to oversee and provide services.

Serving Children Birth through Two Years

Beginning in 1986, with the passage of Public Law 99-457, the federal government adopted legislation designed to address the needs of infants and toddlers with known disabilities or developmental delays, and the needs of their families. The purpose for formulating legislation to serve this population is made clear in Public Law 99-457. Congress found a substantial need to:

(1) enhance the development of infants and toddlers to minimize their potential for development delay,
(2) minimize the educational costs to our society by minimizing the needs for special education services when children reach school age,
(3) minimize the likelihood of institutionalization and maximize potential for independent living,
(4) enhance the capacity of families to meet the special needs of their infants and toddlers with disabilities, and
(5) enhance the capacity of service providers to identify, evaluate, and meet the needs of historically underrepresented populations, particularly minority, low-income, inner city, and rural populations. (P.L. 99-457, 1986, Sec. 671)

Public Law 99-457 and subsequent federal legislation established guidelines for identifying infants and toddlers in need of special services. Infants and toddlers are eligible for services if they (1) are experiencing developmental delays in one or more of the following areas: (a) cognitive; (b) physical, including vision and hearing; (c) communication; (d) social and emotional; (e) adaptive; or (2) have a diagnosed physical or mental condition that has a high probability of resulting in developmental delay (e.g., chromosomal abnormalities; genetic or congenital disorders; severe sensory impairments, including hearing and vision; disorders secondary to exposure to toxic substances, including fetal alcohol syndrome; and severe attachment disorders). States have been empowered to set their own guidelines as to what constitutes a "developmental delay." Furthermore, states may provide services to infants and toddlers who are at risk of having substantial developmental delays if early intervention services are not provided. In defining "at risk" population, states may include well-known biological and environmental conditions (e.g., low birth weight, nutritional deprivation, history of abuse or neglect).

Public law mandates specific policies and procedures for serving infants and toddlers. Public awareness activities have to be initiated by lead agencies that inform the general public of the availability of early intervention services. Once infants and toddlers have been identified as needing special services through interviews, screening, and a variety of assessment measures, a team comprised of the parents and professionals develop an Individual Family Service Plan (IFSP). The IFSP is a written document that contains statements of:

(1) the child's present level of physical, cognitive, communication, social or emotional, and adaptive development,
(2) the needs of the family relative to enhancing the development of their child,
(3) the major outcomes to be achieved by providing services, and the criteria, procedures, and timelines used to determine the degree of progress toward the outcomes,
(4) the specific early intervention services necessary to meet the unique needs of the child,
(5) the natural environment in which early intervention services will be provided,
(6) a statement of projected date of initiation and anticipated duration of services, and
(7) the service coordinator who will be responsible for the implementation of the IFSP.

The IFSP is the cornerstone of early intervention and identifies the type of service (e.g., special instruction, family training, home visits, speech therapy, occupational therapy, psychological services, physical therapy, assistive technology, and other services) and the qualified personnel responsible for providing the service (e.g., physical therapists, occupational therapists, psychologists, social workers, nurses, special educators, and others as necessary) (Donaldson, 1995).

Serving Children Three to School Age

Public Law 94-142, the Education for All Handicapped Children Act, was passed in 1975 and implemented in 1978. This law mandates that all individuals with disabilities, age three to 21 years, must have access to a free, appropriate public education. However, the legislation allowed states not to serve children three to five years if the mandate was incompatible with state law. In 1986, Public Law 99-457 amended P.L. 94-142, and children three to five years were extended the same rights and services (e.g., full public education, due process, court appeals) that were available to school age children. States must now serve preschool children, age three to school age, who are eligible under the categorical areas of mental retardation, hearing impairments, speech or language impairments, visual impairments, serious emotional disturbance, orthopedic impairments, autism, traumatic brain injury, other health impaired, specific learning disability, deaf-blindness, or multiple disabilities and who, because of those impairments, need special education and related services. States, at their discretion, may also include children who are experiencing developmental delays in cognitive development, communication development, social or emotional development, or adaptive development; and who, for that reason, need special education and related services. Once eligible children have been identified through appropriate diagnostic instruments and procedures, a meeting is held with the parents and appropriate professionals to develop an Individual Education Program (IEP) or, for some children transitioning from aged birth through two, programs to review and revise the child's IFSP.

The IEP, like the IFSP, is a written document that provides important information to all parties on the services the child and family will receive. For professionals, the IEP provides information on the child's strengths and current levels of development, the specially designed instruction and related services necessary to meet the goals and objectives established for the child, special materials and intervention strategies, and the method of monitoring child progress. For the family, the IEP explains the services the child and family will receive in language that is easily understood.

Number of Children and Families Birth to School Age Being Served

States have reported a steady increase in the number of children three to school age and birth to three served in programs (U.S. Department of Education, 1997). The number of infants and toddlers receiving services increased 22 percent from 1992 through 1995, to approximately 180,000 children. This accounts for approximately 1.5 percent of all infants and toddlers in the resident population. Children ages two to three continue to represent the majority of children served in this group, accounting for approximately 50 percent of all infants and toddlers receiving services.

The number of preschool children who receive special services has increased 30 percent from 1992 through 1995 to approximately 650,000 children. This exceeded the growth of the general preschool population during this time period (i.e., 8.3 percent). This accounts for approximately 4.5 percent of the general population of this age group. The growth of services to young children reflects the goal of early childhood special education—to enable every child to start school ready to learn (U.S. Department of Education, 1997).

CONTRIBUTIONS OF EARLY CHILDHOOD SPECIAL EDUCATION TO INTERDISCIPLINARY PRACTICE

The interdependence of disciplines serving young children with special needs is the foundation of Early Childhood Special Education (ECSE) and is far different from services provided school age children in need of special services. Multidisciplinary service delivery has always been a central provision of services to children with special needs in schools and evolved from language adopted from P.L. 94-142. Historically, in serving school age students, even with provisions specified in P.L. 94-142, professionals remained independent in assessments and treatments and were affected little by other team members. With the enactment of P.L. 99-457, extending services to children three years to school age, Congress recognized the inherent need for cross-disciplinary collaboration if this age group was to be served appropriately (Bagnato & Neisworth, 1991). Further, much broader interdependence of disciplines was the intent of Congress in legislating services for infants and toddlers (IDEA; P.L. 102-119, 1990; Part C of the Amendments to the Individuals with Disabilities Education Act; P.L. 105-17, 1997). Implementers of services for this age group were directed to design an early intervention system that was "comprehensive, coordinated, multi-disciplinary, [and] interagency" (Section 671 [b][1]; Garrett, Thorp, Behrmann, & Denham, 1998). It was expected that younger children would require services from a far more diverse array of disciplines and service providers, operating from multiple agencies and organizations. The intent of Congress was the development of a system of services that crossed traditional agency and discipline boundaries (Garrett, Thorp, Behrmann, & Denham, 1998) and challenged practitioners to collaborate at both systems development and individual service levels (McGonigel, Woodruff, & Roszmann-Millican, 1994).

At the systems development level, Congress required each state to develop an interagency coordinating council to assist existing state agencies in developing and implementing services for young children. States have extended interagency collaboration to the local level by establishing local interagency coordinating councils. These councils allow parents and professionals to work collaboratively to ensure that adequate and necessary services are available to families and children.

Two distinct levels of service collaboration exist at the individual service level: interagency collaboration and service provider-family collaboration. In interagency collaboration, administrators and service providers from different agencies work together to provide early intervention services. Collaboration is fostered when administrative philosophy encourages professionals to establish relationships with their counterparts at different agencies. Collaboration also is advanced when service providers in different agencies working with the same families share information, resources, and decision-making power (Jeisen, 1996). Interagency agreements are the by products of administrative interagency collaboration. They also formalize responsibilities of agencies in the identification, evaluation, and delivery of services to families and children.

At the service provider-family level, the multifaceted needs of children and families are addressed through the combined efforts of parents and professionals from numerous disciplines. The variety of services that comprise the core of fundable services within early intervention include family training, counseling and home visits, physical therapy, psychological services, occupational therapy, speech pathology and audiology, assistive technology devises and services, medical services (necessary for diagnostic and evaluation services), early identification, screening, and assessment, related health services (as necessary for the child to benefit from early intervention services), vision services, and transportation. The team composition (e.g., special educators, speech pathologists, physical therapists, social workers, physicians) varies and depends on the needs of the child and family (Tuchman, 1996). At the heart of the team composition is the service coordinator. Federal legislation (Part H, P.L. 102-119, 1990; Part C, P.L. 105-17, 1997) requires that each eligible child and the child's family be provided a service coordinator, at the parents' discretion, to assist in the multiple functions of case management (i.e., to ensure all services identified on the IFSP are delivered in a timely manner and to identify additional services that may be of assistance to the family) (Romer & Umbert, 1998).

The team is the vehicle that is able to address the multifaceted needs of the child and family. A team approach has been used historically to plan for and implement services for children with disabilities. The particular feature that characterizes an early intervention team is the common goal of supporting and strengthening the family, as well as addressing the needs of the child (Bailey et al., 1998; Mahoney & Wheeden, 1997; Tuchman, 1996). Other factors that distinguish early childhood teams from school-aged-based teams are the greater number of professionals involved, the style of team collaboration, and the central role parents may assume (Bagnato & Neisworth, 1991). Several models of special education team practices have emerged over the years. Teams that are typically used in early intervention are the multidisciplinary, interdisciplinary, and transdisciplinary teams. Each is unique in its interaction among team members and the methods by which they implement early intervention services. Numerous variables impact upon which team model is adopted. Decisions about which model is employed and how services are rendered depend upon the philosophy of its members, communication between members, available time for team meetings, and responsibilities of its members (Bruder & Bologna, 1993; Woodruff & McGonigel, 1988). Other contributing factors may include environments in which services are delivered (e.g., center-based or home-based), the number of different agencies involved, or the amount of involvement parents desire (Tuchman, 1996). For more information on the multidisciplinary and interdisciplinary team structures, see Chapter 1 of this text. The intent of Congress in passing early childhood special education legislation was a movement from more traditional team models to a transdisciplinary approach.

Transdisciplinary teams are composed of parents and professionals from various disciplines. However, they differ from multidisciplinary and interdisciplinary teams by systematically crossing disciplinary boundaries, sharing and reversing roles in interactions with the child and family, committing to consensus building, and placing the family in the center of the decision-making process (Bagnato & Neisworth, 1991; McGonigel et al., 1994; Tuchman, 1996). The transdisciplinary approach allows for parents and professionals to cross traditional disciplinary boundaries because of a strong commitment to communicate, interact, and collaborate on all facets of the early intervention process. The more familiar team members become with each other's traditional roles and responsibilities, the easier it becomes to develop a common language, understanding, and commitment to shared responsibility in the process. Role release is a central tenant of a transdisciplinary approach. Professionals teach their discipline-specific skills to others and learn new skills from other professionals. Team members believe that by crossing traditional boundaries and learning new skills, intervention is more effective (Tuchman, 1996). Within a transdisciplinary approach there is a strong commitment to consensus building in all areas of assessment, program planning, intervention, and program. The central component of a transdisciplinary approach is the importance of the family in the early intervention process. Families are integral components of the transdisciplinary team and are afforded the degree of involvement they desire in all decisions promulgated by the team.

An *arena assessment* is an example of a transdisciplinary activity. Rather than having a child assessed by numerous professionals in different locations and at different times, an arena assessment allows parents and professionals to gather important information about the child in a naturalistic, less threatening setting. In an arena assessment, team members meet prior to the assessment to agree upon developmental areas to be observed. One team member and/or a parent is responsible for directly interacting with the child while other members of the team observe the child or consult with the parent over the behavior the child is exhibiting. Team members can request certain interactions between the child and individual to elicit certain responses from the child. The important component is that the assessment has been planned by all team members, and all have responsibilities during the assessment process. The arena assessment is a clear way that different disciplines can work toward a common goal.

Although all members of the transdisciplinary team share responsibility for evaluation and program development, interventions are generally carried out by the parents and one service provider, with consultation from other team members. Parent and family members become primary decision-makers and co-interventionists in this approach to service delivery.

Although the transdisciplinary team approach may be considered best practice for infants, toddlers and their families, in light of federal mandates, in reality, the model or models a team incorporates is based on a variety of factors. Whichever model is employed, however, the foremost concern should be the role parents want to play in the decision-making process.

THE ROLES PARENTS TYPICALLY PLAY IN THE OPTIMAL INTERDISCIPLINARY PROVISION OF EARLY CHILDHOOD SPECIAL EDUCATION

With the inception of Part H of IDEA (currently referred to as Part C of the Amendments to the Individuals with Disabilities Act [P.L. 105-17; 1997]), a significant shift occurred concerning the relationship between parents and professionals (Winton, 1994; Turnbull & Turnbull, 1996). In the past, the child or the mother-child dyad was the focus of professional interaction. Today, professionals understand there are issues beyond the child that must be addressed to effectively serve children (Nineteenth Annual Report to Congress, 1997). The needs and strengths of the family, as well as the child, are important components which are brought into the process when developing educational programs to assist children and families.

The shift toward a family systems approach was stimulated by three developments since the 1970s (Mahoney & Bella, 1998). First, assumptions presented by Bronfenbrenner (1979) stressed that parenting behavior is influenced by forces both external and internal to the family system and that the manner in which parents interacted with their children played a critical role in children's development. Second, research began to reveal that positive intervention effects occurred when programs made significant efforts to work directly with parents (Dunst, Trivette, & Deal, 1988). Last, the professional community began to understand that, although parents had the most influence on their child's development in the early years, there were significant social and psychological burdens placed on parents and families that made it difficult to raise a child with disabilities (Dunst, Trivette, & Jordy, 1997; Harris & McHale, 1989).

By acknowledging the unique financial, social and psychological stresses placed on families that may weaken the family unit and have critical consequences for the long-term care and development of children with disabilities, sustaining and supporting families became as important a goal as the developmental outcomes of the child. Enabling parents to maximize their abilities and competencies at promoting the development and well-being of their children became the fundamental concern that chartered the shift from a professionally-driven service model to a family systems service model in early childhood intervention.

Hanson and Lynch (1995) underscore the rationale for a shift to a family systems perspective by identifying several factors. Parents and significant caregivers are the most important people in the child's life. It is the parents' right to make decisions regarding their child. Parents have legal rights for input and decision-making in the educational process. Parental input and carryover in the home are essential for optimal effects of early intervention efforts. Early intervention can assist parents to experience positive relationships with their children and support parents to keep their children in their homes. Early services can provide information and support to parents to use community resources more effectively. Active involvement and input can ensure more fully coordinated services. Finally, parental involvement in programs may be more economical. With a shift toward a family systems approach in early intervention, additional expectations may be placed on parents as they are afforded a greater role in the early intervention process.

As the shift toward greater decision-making power residing with parents continues, many parents are unprepared to serve the executive parent function. Parents have not been trained as recruiters, hirers, firers, advocates, consumers, coordinators, or professionals (Begun, 1996). In many cases parents do not have the information to serve in those capacities. The informational needs of parents continue to impede their ability to effectively make decisions about service options for their child. Furthermore, the informational needs may differ with regards to gender of the parent, race, socioeconomic status, and educational level (Gowen, Christy, & Sparling, 1993; Sontag & Schacht, 1994). There appears to be strong evidence of the need for early intervention professionals to provide information to parents as a program outcome, and more specifically, information about what services are available and how the system works.

Information begets involvement and parental contribution in the early intervention process and tends to empower the parent and enhance optimism regarding the child's opportunities. An example follows of a parent who enrolled her son in an early intervention program and was confused about the role she could play in the child's education. With only a high school education, she felt inadequate and self-conscious about her lack of knowledge regarding her child's disability.

Brad was born with Down syndrome. He is two years old and has trouble doing just about everything. I didn't get services for him right away because I didn't know that I could. So I kept him at home with me until he was 18 months old. Now he is in an early intervention program and he likes it a lot. He doesn't talk yet, but he gets excited when the bus comes to pick him up. He attends the program all day, five days a week, which is good for me because I work. At first I thought the program would take care of Brad's education, but I was starting to feel I wasn't doing enough. I spoke with his teacher, and she invited me to a team meeting. I agreed to come, but at the last minute, I didn't go. I couldn't imagine sitting in a room with all those educated people and wasn't sure what I was supposed to do with Brad, anyway. The teacher asked why I didn't show up and I finally told her I was just scared to death. We talked for awhile, and she told me I was an expert about my son and that no one knew him as well as I did. Then she told me to call a parents group for families of children who had Down syndrome. That was the best advice I ever received. I went to the parents group meeting and listened to parents talk about how afraid they were at first and how dumb they felt. But they had to get over it because they knew that the child would do better in school, and they would feel better if they were involved. I go to the team meetings now. The professionals are wonderful and make me feel like I'm doing something to help Brad. I don't understand everything that they say, but I know enough to ask if I don't. I am grateful for the help and I am grateful because I can help my son.

Most parents are very interested in their child's care and educational activities. They need to feel they can do something to help their child. Empowering families helps to foster a subtle shift from professionally driven services to an equal partnership between parents and professionals. Early intervention appears to be most effective when the focus of the parent-professional relationship is on empowering families. Involvement and parental contribution in the early intervention process tends to empower the parent, and enhance optimism regarding the child's opportunities. Professionals who provide early intervention services should encourage parents' involvement through building relationships. Professionals should establish reciprocal relationships, listen and respond in a nonbiased manner, and integrate and adapt information obtained to assist with interventions. A father of a young girl with spina bifida shares this experience on providing information that helped assist with more meaningful interventions.

Sarah was born with spina bifida. She is unable to walk and also has trouble using her hands, so she was unable to adjust to crutches. She attends an

Easter Seals program five days a week. The first year she was in the program, I was not involved with the early intervention team. The special educator would report what they talked about, but I always felt left out. And sometimes they would try to implement treatment activities that I knew Sarah was not going to do. I complained long and hard and was finally invited to a team meeting. The team leader was nice enough, but some of the other members were a little impatient with my presence. The occupational therapist, who was trying to improve Sarah's ability to use her hands, asked what I thought about the exercises and activities that were used. I took a deep breath (I was quite intimidated) and told her that Sarah couldn't do them. They were too hard for her, and if they were too hard, she wouldn't try. I told her that Sarah was very aware of her limitations and the worse thing in the world was to try something that was too difficult. I said it was better to take little steps with Sarah, not big steps, and she would improve a little bit at a time. You could hear a pin drop. I thought I had blown it. Finally, the occupational therapist said, "I'm glad you told us that. We should have had you talk with us a long time ago." She gave me a list of things to do at home and invited me to the next meeting. I feel much more involved with Sarah's education, instead of as an observer. And it turns out that I am a pretty good teacher.

Involving fathers is an important component of early childhood special education services. Until recently, little research had been done on the role fathers play in this process. Pearl (1993) commented that even though fathers may not participate as actively as mothers in the care of young children, their outlook and acceptance is essential to the family's response to early intervention services. Fathers have reported only half as many family needs as mothers (Bailey & Simeonsson, 1988) and less stress than mothers as a result of group discussions (Upsur, 1991). Yet fathers also feel more pessimistic and less empowered to make a difference on their child's behalf (Vadasy, Fewell, Greenberg, Dermond, & Meyer, 1986). Strategies to facilitate a father's involvement have begun to be developed. The Association for the Care of Children's Health found that fathers are more likely to attend meetings if goals, times, and meetings are clearly specified and that support meetings will be responsive to issues they themselves have raised (Bowe, 1995).

Siblings, as well as fathers, may have specific issues related to a brother or sister with a disability. They may resent the attention given the child with disabilities, or they may feel as though they have been forced prematurely into adult roles (Bowe, 1995). It is important for parents to realize these feelings exist and identify times for meaningful interactions with those siblings. It also may be necessary to seek out support groups for siblings without disabilities so they can share their concerns with other siblings with similar experiences. Support groups increase siblings' knowledge of disabilities and help to identify strengths of different family members.

There is continuing evolvement toward families assuming a greater role in the processes involved in early childhood special education. This will intensify when professionals have the skills to enable and empower families, and parents have the information they need to become equal participants in the process.

TYPICAL PARENT QUESTIONS/COMMENTS FOR EARLY CHILDHOOD SPECIAL EDUCATION

Current practices in Early Childhood Special Education focus on individualizing services for families and basing the efforts of the team on the expressed needs of family members. However, there remain some areas that continue to raise parental concern. The following are some of the questions that were asked by parents on the parent survey.

Many professionals are patronizing and talk down to parents. How can we promote an atmosphere that respects parents' rights to be part of the decision-making process, based upon a holistic approach including religion, culture and lifestyle?

It is important to remember that professionals are concerned about their changing roles. Professionals continue to feel more competent in working with children than they do working with parents. Although the legislative focus is on addressing the needs of families, professionals themselves are uncertain of their skills in family-centered practices. As professionals become trained and experienced in a family-centered practice, they will be more confident in their role within this new approach of working with families.

Fundamentally, it is important for parents to become knowledgeable of the specific rights they have in the early intervention and special education process. These rights have to be presented to parents by agencies or school personnel in written form, in language they can understand. Parents have specific rights in all phases of the early intervention and special education process, including assessment of child and family strengths and needs, program planning, and the setting in which a program is to be offered. Parents have the right to question, challenge, or refuse any actions proposed by an agency or school in relation to the education of their child.

Issues regarding cultural differences, lifestyles, and religion should be considered in all phases of the intervention process, from initial contacts to setting outcomes for the child and family. Cultural sensitivity and competence is an important component of all interactions between families and service agency personnel. Following family-centered principles is an important first step. Various professionals may need to modify their written policies and procedures to be representative of culturally sensitive issues. Self-study programs are available to agencies to assess their practices of providing culturally sensitive services. Rosin (1996) elaborates a four step process for practitioners to strengthen cultural competence: (1) exploring one's own cultural attitudes, values, and practices; (2) exploring some of the sources of family diversity, such as culture, family structure, socioeconomic status, and parents who have disabilities; (3) understanding the barriers encountered by families in gaining access to and participating in early intervention; and (4) developing early intervention services that are responsive to diverse families. Professionals should be sensitive to the differences in families regarding communication style, decision-making, and the need or willingness to seek assistance from individuals outside the family circle (Hanson & Lynch, 1995). Parents should feel free to assist the professional in understanding the culture of the family unit. The professional's task is to accept the practices of the families as valid and important, although they may be different from those practiced by the dominant culture in that geographical area (Hanson & Lynch, 1995).

Ask questions and seek answers. Information is an important ally.

Why do some professionals avoid labels in favor of terms like "developmental delay?" Shouldn't you call it like you see it?

Many of the same reasons are used for identifying children as developmentally delayed in the birth through two years of age and the three years to school age groups. In the birth through two years age group, if a child does not have a known physical or mental condition which has a high probability of resulting in developmental delay, Part C regulations specify the developmental areas that are to be included in states' definitions of developmental delay. States are expressing criteria for delay in various ways, such as: (1) difference between chronological age and actual performance level expressed as a percentage of chronological age, (2) delay expressed as performance at a certain number of months below chronological age, (3) delay as indicated by standard deviation below the mean on a norm referenced instrument, or (4) delay indicated by atypical development or observed atypical behaviors. The amount of delay a child must exhibit to receive services also varies between states. The most prominent reasons given for the use of a noncategorical label (i.e., developmental delay) is that there is a lack of reliable and valid assessment instruments for this age group and infants and toddlers do not fit the eligibility criteria established for school-age children. Young children's development is also not uniform. For example, some children may present global developmental delays at 18 months and after a year of intervention may just have speech/language delays.

For preschool children, it makes sense to provide eligibility options stated in terms of "developmental" rather than "educational." Existing categorical definitions for school-age children include three criteria for eligibility: (1) presence of a documented disability (e.g., specific learning disabled, mentally disabled, behaviorally-emotionally impaired); (2) which adversely affects a child's educational performance; and (3) require(s) special instruction. These criteria pose problems in the identification process for young children. Difficulties in the assessment of young children may make the results of tests unreliable. It is also difficult to document adverse effects of a disability on educational performance because preschoolers have no previous educational experience. What is known is the child's developmental status. There may be concerns about the application of a categorical label when a child reaches school age after the child has been identified as developmentally delayed through preschool. It is important for parents to understand that a developmental delay label is temporary and that when children reach school age, a new categorical label will be applied if they are in continued need of special education services. This should not be as great a concern if parents are appraised of this fact early during their interactions with the special education process during preschool.

Placing a categorical label on a child has also become a major issue. Some individuals believe labels affect a teacher's expectations, and thus may have a negative impact on the child's educational progress.

How hard should I push for my child's inclusion in a regular preschool setting? He has been described as having moderate disabilities, yet he is social and interested in others.

There are benefits to preschool integration for preschoolers with disabilities. McCormick (1994) identifies four arguments for placing preschoolers in inclusive settings: (1) inclusive experiences are the primary means children with special needs can learn the ways in the normal world, (2) noninclusive settings provide limited socialization experiences, (3) young children with disabilities must have continuous opportunities to observe and imitate normal same-age peers, and (4) inclusive settings encourage positive attitudes and awareness that children with disabilities are more similar than different from their peers without disabilities.

Cole, Mills, Dale, and Jenkins (1991) found that lower performing preschoolers made greater developmental gains in segregated setting, whereas higher performing children with disabilities made greater gains in integrated settings. Gains have also been reported in the social domain when students with disabilities are placed in inclusive settings (Edmister & Ekstrand, 1987).

Most importantly, federal and state laws mandate a continuum of educational placements for children. A variety of placement options should be available to children in order to meet their individual needs. This means an inclusive setting may be an option, but other non-inclusive settings should also be considered if they more appropriately meet the child's goals and objectives. Parents should always advocate for their child to be placed in the least restrictive environment that meets the individual needs of their child.

Dr. Schulz's Response:

The authors' response that parents should insist on the least restrictive environment that meets the individual needs of their child is a wise and important one. Many of us as parents insist on total inclusion without considering the benefits of alternatives. I am reminded of a young girl whose parents I have known for years, and whose progress through school I have observed and been concerned about.

Susan has Down syndrome. She is attractive, social and verbal. Her parents have insisted that she remain totally in the regular classroom from kindergarten through graduation from high school. Periodically, special educators have urged her parents to consider at least part-time placement of Susan in a vocationally-oriented class for students with moderate retardation. As a parent and a professional, I was asked for my opinion by the parents. They were surprised and displeased that I agreed with the educators and they refused to make a change.

Susan struggled with reading programs, with math beyond her abilities and science and social studies that had no meaning for her. Although she was socially accepted and competent in the early grades, the gap of understanding and communication between her and her peers broadened as she grew older.

Meanwhile, students in the class for those with moderate retardation were learning job skills, homemaking skills, and useful communication. Part of their program included working in sheltered and community work settings.

Susan has graduated from school and stays at home without promise or expectation of community integration. While this is an extreme example, it is a real one and emphasizes the importance of exploring options and looking to future needs of the child.

CASE EXAMPLE

Jill's developmental history was typical of children born prematurely. She was delivered by Cesarean section at 38 weeks gestation because of respiratory distress, which required oxygen. Seizures occurred within 24 hours, requiring treatment. Jill was hospitalized for two weeks at which time Jill's parents were told she may be "at risk" for later developmental delays.

Jill showed steady physical growth during her first two years. However, the parents were increasingly concerned about the number of middle ear infections, low muscle tone, and poor eye-hand coordination their daughter seemed to have.

At two years of age, Jill preferred to point or gesture to communicate and had a ten word vocabulary. When Jill did speak, many basic sounds were unintelligible. She was having difficulty using a spoon for feeding. Although Jill was walking independently, she was having difficulty climbing up on furniture or going down stairs with help. She always preferred to crawl down the stairs backward.

Her parents became increasingly concerned when they compared abilities to an older sibling. They talked to their pediatrician who was able to locate county-wide early intervention services.

They were initially very impressed with their first meeting with an early intervention educational consultant. The individual they met with took all the time necessary to answer all the questions Jill's parents had concerning their daughter's delays and the sequence and scope of services that may be available to Jill through early intervention services.

The following week, an arena assessment was scheduled at Jill's home. A few days prior to arriving at the home, the occupational therapist and speech/language pathologist called Jill's parents to introduce themselves and discuss the procedure for the arena assessment and to be clear on the concerns of Jill's parents. On the day of the assessment, three early interventionists arrived (educational consultant, speech/language pathologist, and occupational therapist) and held a short meeting with the parents to discuss some specific behaviors they wanted to elicit from Jill during the assessment. The assessment provided very good information on Jill's language, cognitive, and motor skills. Following the assessment, the parents and interventionists initially met to discuss some of their finding relative to Jill's performance and to elicit any concerns or help the parents may want with family issues.

The following week all members met with the parents at their home and developed an IFSP that addressed specific objectives in the areas of language, fine motor, and cognitive skills. The parents decided that they wanted to be the primary interventionists with their child and requested that the speech/language pathologist be the co-interventionist, since language development was their greatest concern at the moment. It was agreed that the speech/language pathologist would act as the case manager and be responsible for transferring the interventions from the occupational therapist and educational consultant to the parents. It was decided that the case manager would also address the family needs that were identified on the IFSP.

Jill's parents were pleased that not only were their concerns heard, but they were able to participate actively on their daughter's behalf. They were made to feel as though they were the most important members of the team. The parents' active involvement increased their confidence in their abilities to help Jill achieve her potential.

Over the past decade, numerous changes have begun to occur in the field of Early Childhood Special Education. Services for young children with special needs have gone from child-centered programs to family-centered programs, from segregated settings to inclusionary settings, from programs designed by professionals to programs designed by parents and professionals. The most important change, however, is the focus on strengthening families of children with disabilities through interdisciplinary relationships between parents and professionals.

Editors' Note:

   Oren provides a cogent argument for the use of transdisciplinary teaming when providing services to infants, toddlers and their families. We agree that the transdisciplinary model, as described in Chapter 1 and again by Oren, is thought to reflect best practice with this population. That said, the editors caution against entering a transdisciplinary teaming relationship unless all team members embrace the tenets of transdisciplinary practice (e.g., role release, family centeredness...).

REFERENCES

Bagnato, S. T., & Neisworth, J. T. (1991). *Assessment for early intervention: Best practices for professionals.* New York: Guilford Press.

Bailey, D. B., McWilliam, R. A., Darkes, L., Hebbler, K., Simeonsson, R., Spiker, D., & Wagner, M. (1998). Family outcomes in early intervention: A framework for program evaluation and efficacy research. *Exceptional Children, 64* (3), 313-328.

Bailey, D. B., & Simeonsson, R. (1988). *Family assessment in early intervention.* Columbus, OH: Charles E. Merrill.

Begun, A. L. (1996). Family systems and family centered practices. In P. Rosin, A. Whitehead, L. Tuchman, G. Jesien, A. Begun, & L. Irwin (Eds.), *Partnerships in family centered care* (pp. 33-63). Baltimore: Paul H Brookes.

Bowe, F. (1995). *Birth to five: Early childhood special education.* New York: Delmar.

Bronfenbrenner, U. (1979). *The ecology of human development.* Cambridge, MA: Harvard University Press.

Bruder, M. B., & Bologna, T. (1993). Collaboration and service coordination for effective early intervention. In W. Brown, S. K. Thurman, & L. F. Pearl (Eds.), *Family centered early intervention with infants and toddlers: Innovative cross-disciplinary approaches* (pp. 103-127). Baltimore: Paul H. Brookes.

Cole, K. N., Mills, P. E., Dale, P. S., & Jenkins, J. R. (1991). Effects of preschool intervention for children with disabilities. *Exceptional Children, 58,* 36-45.

Donaldson, S. (1995). Comprehensive early intervention program resources. Unpublished master's thesis, The Pennsylvania State University, State College.

Dunst, C. J., Trivette, C. M., & Deal. (1988). *Enabling and empowering families: Principles and guidelines for practice.* Cambridge MA: Brookline Books.

Dunst, C. J., Trivette, C. M., & Jodry, W. (1997). Influences on social support on children with disabilities and their families. In M. J. Guralnick (Ed.), *Effectiveness of early intervention* (pp. 499-522). Baltimore: Paul H. Brookes .

Edminister, P., & Ekstrand, R. E. (1987). Preschool programming: Legal end educational issues. *Exceptional Children, 54,* 130-136.

Education of the Handicapped Act amendments of 1986, PL 99-457. (October, 8, 1986). Title 20, U.S.C. 1400 et seq. *U.S. Statutes at Large,* 100, 1145-1177.

Garrett, J., Thorpe, E., Behrmann, M., & Denham, S. (1998). The impact of early intervention legislation: Local perspectives. *Topics in Early Childhood Special Education, 17* (2), 165-184.

Gowen, J. W., Christy, D. S., & Sparling, J. (1993). Informational needs of parents of young children with special needs. *Journal of Early Intervention, 17* (2), 194-210.

Hanson, J. H., & Lynch, E. W. (1995). *Early intervention: Implementing child and family services for infants and toddlers who are at risk or disabled.* Austin, TX: Pro-Ed.

Individuals with Disabilities Act (IDEA) of 1990, P.L. 101-476 (October 30, 1990). Title 20, U.S.C. 1400 et seq.

Individuals with Disabilities Education Act Amendments of 1991, P.L. 102-119, (October, 7, 1991). Title 20, U.S.C. 1400 et seq: *U.S. Statutes at Large,* 105, 587-608.

Jesien, G. (1996). Interagency collaboration: What, why, and with whom. In P. Rosin, A. Whitehead, L. Tuchman, G. Jesien, A. Begun, & L. Irwin (Eds.), *Partnerships in family centered care* (pp. 201-224). Baltimore: Paul H Brookes.

Mahoney, G., & Bella, T. (1998). An examination of the effects of family-centered early intervention on child and family outcomes. *Topics in Early Childhood Special Education, 18* (2), 83-94.

Mahoney, G., & Wheeden, A. C. (1997). Parent-child interactions-the foundations for family-centered early intervention practice: A response to Baird and Peterson. *Topics in Early Childhood Special Education, 17* (2) 165-184.

McCormick, L. (1994). Infants and young children with special needs. In N. G. Haring, L. McCormick, & T. G. Haring (Eds.), *Exceptional Children and Youth (6th ed.* (pp. 86-112). Upper Saddle River, NJ: Merrill/Prentice Hall.

McGonigel, M., Woodruff, G., & Roszmann-Millican, L. (1994). The transdisciplinary model: A model for family-centered early intervention. In L. L. Johnson, R. J. Gallagher, M. S. LaMontague, J. B. Jordon. P. Hutinger, J. Gallagher, & M. B. Karnes (Eds.), *Meeting early intervention challenges: Issues from birth to three* (pp. 95-131). Baltimore: Paul Brookes.

Pearl, L. (1993). Providing family-centered early intervention. In W. Brown, S. Thurman, & L. Pearl (Eds.), *Family centered early intervention with infants and toddlers: Innovative cross-disciplinary approaches* (pp. 81-101). Baltimore: Paul H. Brookes.

Romer, E., & Umbert, J. (1998). The effects of family-centered service coordination: A social validity study. *Journal of Early Intervention, 21* (2), 95-110.

Rosin, P. (1996). The diverse American family. In P. Rosin, A. Whitehead, L. Tuchman, G. Jesien, A. Begun, & L. Irwin (Eds.), *Partnerships in family centered care* (pp. 3-32). Baltimore: Paul H Brookes.

Sixteenth Annual Report to Congress on the Implementation of the Individuals with disabilities Education Act (1994). Washington, D.C: U.S. Department of Education.

Sontag, J., & Schacht, R. (1994). An ethnic comparison of participation and information needs in early intervention. *Exceptional Children, 60* (5), 422-433.

Tuchmann, L. I. (1996). The team and models of teaming. In P. Rosin, A. Whitehead, L. Tuchman, G. Jesien, A. Begun, & L. Irwin (Eds.), *Partnerships in family centered care* (pp. 119-143). Baltimore: Paul H Brookes.

Turnbull, A. P., & Turnbull, H. R. (1996). *Families, professionals, and exceptionality.* Upper Saddle River, NJ: Merrill.

Upsur, C. (1991). Mothers' and fathers' ratings of the benefits of early intervention services. *Journal of Early Intervention, 15,* 345-357.

Vadasy, P., Fewell, R., Greenberg, M., Dermond, N., & Meyer, D. (1986). Follow-up evaluation of the effects of involvement in the fathers program. *Topics in Early Childhood Special Education, 6* (1), 16-31.

Winton, P. J. (1994). Families of children with disabilities. In W. G. Haring, L. Mccormick, & T. G. Haring (Eds.), *Exceptional children and youth* (6th ed.) (pp. 502-525). New York: Merrill.

Woodruff, G., & McGonigel, M. (1988). Early intervention team approaches: The transdisciplinary model. In J. Gordon, P. Huntinger, M. Karnes, & J. Gallagher (Eds.), *Early childhood special education* (pp. 163-181). Reston, VA: Council for Exceptional Children.

Chapter 12

SPECIAL EDUCATION

STEVE COLSON AND KATHLEEN CARR

A key person delivering services to students with special needs is the classroom teacher, both in the general education setting and in the special class. These professionals begin their work during the assessment process and continue throughout the intervention stages. They are also important in assisting other related service providers to ensure a collaborative effort. This chapter will present the major responsibilities and roles of the special education teacher, as well as the contributions of special education to interdisciplinary practice. Additionally, the roles parents typically play in working optimally with teachers will be addressed. Finally, solutions to specific questions from parents regarding special education are discussed, and a case study is presented.

MAJOR ROLES AND RESPONSIBILITIES OF SPECIAL EDUCATORS

Although most general classroom teachers have some beginning level knowledge about teaching students with special needs, it is really the special education teacher who assesses needs and plans lessons to help a student master curriculum content. Related service providers such as speech-language pathologists, occupational/physical therapists, and social workers provide support to the individual student and the teacher to facilitate success in the classroom. The teacher has the major role in delivering instruction and providing continuity among other professionals on the team.

Special education teachers go through a comprehensive training program (frequently at the graduate level) to learn about child development and how to meet the needs of diverse learners. Since teachers are trained about specific laws regarding special education, they are often the first resource parents can turn to for information about the Individuals with Disabilities Education Act (IDEA).

P.L. 94-142, the Individuals with Disabilities Education Act, was passed in 1975 because it was found that millions of students with disabilities were not being served adequately in our schools. P.L. 94-142 periodically undergoes reauthorization and amendments to respond to changing needs. Although it has been amended several times, two amendments are particularly significant.

First, in 1983 and again in 1986, Congress amended IDEA to provide for early childhood special education. Services specific to this amendment are discussed at length in Chapter 11 of this book. Second, although IDEA provided educational and related services for individuals with disabilities while they were in school, over time it became clear that more help was needed in the transition from school to working and living in the adult world. Thus, Congress amended the law in 1983 and again in 1986 to ensure that students ages sixteen and older would have an education geared to helping them become independent and productive and ready to be included in the mainstream of American life (Turnbull, Turnbull, Shank, & Leal, 1999).

The implementation of IDEA is a shared responsibility among all team members having diagnostic, intervention, or administrative input into the planning process for each student with a disability. Each team member (e.g., the parents, the psychologist, the speech-language pathologist, the social worker, the building administrator) brings forth a unique set of professional abilities to the decision-making process. All members of the diagnostic and planning team should be trained in interdisciplinary methods of role sharing and collaborative consultation. This interdisciplinary approach brings the talents of all of the team members together in an atmosphere of mutual respect and with the desire to serve all of the needs of each individual student.

IDEA attempts to provide a free appropriate public education to every student with a disability, no matter how severe. Six major principles define the parameters of the key phrase *free appropriate public education.* The special educator has a major role in seeing that each of these principles is adhered to. These six principles include zero reject (inclusion in a program of appropriate services), nondiscriminatory evaluation, appropriate education, least restrictive environment, procedural due process, and parent and student participation.

Zero Reject

In essence, the principle of Zero Reject states that a public school cannot deny educational services to any student regardless of the nature or severity of the disability or multiple disabilities. Many special education teachers are trained to instruct students with specific types of disabilities. Parents can always inquire about a teacher's training and his or her experience with other students with the same disability. The special educator should be a first-line advocate in referring students for evaluation and making sure that all children with disabilities are afforded appropriate educational opportunities, regardless of their multiple needs or the severity or complexity of those needs.

Nondiscriminatory Evaluation

All students are entitled to a fair evaluation leading to an appropriate education. Evaluation is performed to document the characteristics of a disability and to help plan instruction in both the general and special classroom. Teachers, psychologists, and other related service personnel assess students for special needs. Special educators are often instrumental in taking information from related service providers and incorporating it into the student's program of instruction. Evaluation will document areas of strength and concern. The term "relative strength" is used to describe a strength for an individual learner rather than comparing that student to others without disabilities. The term "weakness" is not appropriate and parents should discourage this term both in discussions with the team and on any written documentation.

Each school district has developed its own curriculum to document what is taught at each grade level or in each specific content course. Special educators have access to this curriculum skills sequence and use it to help determine the necessary modifications for including a student with special needs in an individual activity. Parents can request a copy of the general education curriculum and ask for a detailed lesson plan that shows how modifications will take place and be evaluated. Special educators have unique skills in knowing how the child's needs fit in the regular curriculum and can help other educators develop appropriate inclusion opportunities.

Appropriate Education

After the interdisciplinary team has determined a student is eligible for special education services, a teaching program is developed for each individual student. This document is referred to as the Individual Education Program (more commonly referred to as IEP). The IEP lists the present level of performance across several different areas of development. Development areas typically include statements about a student's current cognitive (intellectual, problem-solving, and adaptive abilities), academic (reading, written expression and mathematics), social/emotional (peer and family relationships), and language (both receptive and expressive) skills. For preschool children, this type of document is referred to as an Individualized Family Service Plan (IFSP). For more on IFSPs, see Chapter 11.

Specific goals and objectives are outlined using this information. Goals are long-term statements comprised of short-term steps (objectives) that are observable and measurable. For example, a long-term goal could state "Maria will increase her skills in addition." Short-term objectives under this goal could include "Maria will add one-, two-, or three-digit numbers without regrouping," and "Maria will add two-digit numbers with regrouping in the one's place."

A long-range goal could be in place for several months or the entire school year, depending on the student. Short-term objectives are specifically designed to document gains for all involved in this process—the parents, the teachers, and the student. If gains cannot be documented, individual objectives need to be altered. For example, if a student's goal of counting orally to 100 is not met within several months, then perhaps the goal could be broken down more specifically into manageable steps, such as "Maria will count to 25 without prompting." Once this short-term objective is met, then a new objective is taught, building upon this previously learned skill. Parents should ask for several objectives under each goal.

Special educators will be able to lead the team discussion in how related service needs (e.g., language and motor therapy goals) can be infused with the ongoing curriculum in the classroom. Special educators can help insure that the student's needs are listed on the IEP and that specific professionals are identified as service providers. Of course, multiple professionals can work on similar goals.

Least Restrictive Environment

All students with disabilities need to have their instruction with other students who do not have disabilities as much as possible. This decision is made after the IEP is developed by the school's interdisciplinary team. The place where a student is taught is not determined first. Students' individual needs guide the creation of the IEP which guides the school team in determining where those needs will be met.

Most students with disabilities will be included with their nondisabled peers for activities such as art, music and physical education. Some, or most, students will be included for other typical classroom activities in reading, math, and writing. The special educator can help lead a team discussion about the possible benefits of inclusion in various parts of the school day and can even help troubleshoot cases in which another staff member may be reluctant to include a student with special needs. In situations where there is resistance from other team members, the special educator can help model modifications and work with the building administrator in ensuring that a professional trained in special education techniques is available to other team members on an as-needed basis.

Procedural Due Process

IDEA clearly states that parents must agree to the school's findings regarding eligibility, IEP development, and classroom placement. When parents do not agree, they have the right to due process. Parents need to be apprised of their due process rights under IDEA. An advocate also may be useful in the mediation of disagreements.

One important role of special educators will be to remind the principal or other administrators about due process procedures. In-service opportunities often provide the special educator with current information about due process. The special educator, in turn, can inform administrators about specific aspects of due process and how it is implemented in the district. The special educator can also update other team members on current legal decisions and changes in state or federal regulations.

Parent and Student Participation

Parents are integral members of the team. Under IDEA parents have the right to inspect and review all of their child's educational records; have an independent evaluation made of their child; receive written notice of any change in the identification, evaluation, or placement of their child or any change in a child's individual education program; receive an impartial due process hearing if they disagree with the school's decision; and participate equally with school personnel in developing, reviewing, and revising their child's IEP.

Most of these decisions are made with the general and special education teachers working collaboratively with parents. The teacher should be the first person to contact when parents have a question about the education of their child. Since the teacher has direct contact with the student and can implement changes quickly, this should be the primary step in mediating disagreements. If the classroom teacher cannot make changes, or is unwilling to make changes, then the entire interdisciplinary team should be convened to discuss options. It will be helpful for parents to ask for an administrator to be present, especially a special education supervisor. This supervisor typically has the authority to approve IEP changes.

Of course, the responsibility for implementing the parent participation part of IDEA must ultimately fall to the parents. However, special educators can help make parental involvement pleasant and collaborative. The teacher can help set the tone in written and oral communication that is child-focused and respectful. It would be best practice for teachers to build a long term relationship with each family. A positive outcome would be a more unified team where the parent is a valued member and parental concerns are treated with respect. The teacher can be present when there are parental issues with other team members, in the spirit of wanting to make sure the child's needs are met throughout the day.

CONTRIBUTIONS OF SPECIAL EDUCATORS TO INTERDISCIPLINARY PRACTICE

Special educators contribute to interdisciplinary practice in myriad ways. Three major contributions are discussed briefly below.

A significant contribution of Special Education to interdisciplinary practice is peer education. This may include educating the team specific to IDEA. Unfortunately, many team members will not know the six principles described earlier in this chapter. This can be disconcerting given the roles played by professionals other than special educators in evaluation and treatment planning for school-aged children. When team members are unclear about IDEA or other laws, the special educator should provide guidelines specific to the laws and their provisions. This can occur as a part of regular in-service activities. Special educators may also find themselves educating their peers specific to various disabilities and their impact on learning and development. Again, efforts in this regard can occur as a part of in-service activities.

Special educators also contribute to interdisciplinary practice by functioning as a liaison between parents and families, regular educators, and other team members. Because the special educator is uniquely positioned at the hub of service delivery, he or she often receives information from varied sources. The effective dissemination of this information is critical to effective team functioning for the child. For example, conveying a parent's concern that their child is not well may alter assessment plans of other professionals. The role as a liaison is often formalized by the special educator being identified as the team's case coordinator.

Finally, special educators contribute to interdisciplinary practice in the role of child/family advocate. Because they are involved in the total care of the child (e.g., the generation and implementation of the IEP or IFSP), special educators can advocate for children's needs across disciplinary lines. For example, they can contact related service personnel about needs identified by the team but unmet by a specific team member. Child advocacy for the special educator is a natural byproduct of case coordination.

THE ROLES PARENTS TYPICALLY PLAY IN THE OPTIMAL INTERDISCIPLINARY SERVICE PROVISION OF SPECIAL EDUCATION

Parents are vital members of the special education team because no one knows a child as well as the parents. This knowledge can provide other team members with valuable keys to assist in developing plans to help students reach their potential.

Parents can help teachers in several specific and unique ways. First, parents can serve as advocates for their child. Learning about the school system's procedures regarding students with special needs will increase the chances for success in this role. A good place for parent advocates to begin is by requesting a copy of their local school system's procedures and regulations for special education.

Parents also can help teachers by "telling their story." Each family will bring a unique story with them. The telling of this story is a good beginning for working with teachers. Schedule an informal conference to share your child's history and your family story. Be sure to include your child's likes and dislikes, fears, joys, strengths, and areas to target for improvement. It would also be helpful to let the classroom teachers know how your child learns best. For example, is your child a visual learner or an auditory learner? Would it be helpful to limit stimulating factors surrounding the child? Optimally, this sharing would occur at the beginning of a new school year or placement setting. A set of useful questions to ask at your child's school team meeting are listed in Table 12-1. You may want to copy questions and give them to the team a week or so before the meeting to ensure that the professionals have time to gather the necessary information.

Many teachers solicit parents' assistance through the creation of a journal of their child's learning history. Journaling can be both motivating and fun for the child and useful to the child's teachers. The journal could include copies of skills the child has mastered (these would also be available on previous IEPs), samples of the child's work, outside evaluations, and photographs of the child functioning outside the school in family and community settings. For children with complex and multiple needs it might be helpful to have parents provide a brief written synthesis for each teacher. Each professional should have a copy of this summary. This can maximize chances that important information about a child is known by all the members of the interdisciplinary team. It is vital that any health concerns and medications/ treatments are documented.

Table 12-1

COMMON QUESTIONS TO ASK YOUR CHILD'S SPECIAL EDUCATION AND GENERAL EDUCATION TEACHERS

1. What tests were used to document the characteristics of my child's disability?
2. How are these results used to help you create long-term goals and short term objectives for my child?
3. How will you document progress on each of these objectives? How frequently will you collect data to document growth (once a week, once a month, on every activity)?
4. What special materials and methods will you use to help my child master these current goals and objectives? Why did you choose these materials over others?
5. What criteria are you using to determine how much time my child can spend in the general education classroom? How will you document that her special needs are being met in that setting? When will we come together again as a team to discuss if this arrangement is successful?
6. Have you (or any of the other team members) had experience working with other students similar to our child?
7. What can we as parents do at home to help meet my child's goals? Can we volunteer our time to come to school and help?
8. When we have a question regarding our child's education, the federal and state laws/regulations, or other related matters, who should be our first contact person (classroom teacher, case manager, principal, director of special services)?
9. How does my child relate to peers in both the special education and general education classrooms? How can we promote social skills at home and in the community?
10. Do you have a school organization of parents of children with and without special needs that we can join? If not, how could we go about organizing a group?

Finally, parents should also keep a paper trail of all meetings they attend. This log should document the date of each meeting, the names and roles of each participant and each meeting's purpose and outcomes. Table 12-2 shows a sample form that can be used to document the discussion of a team meeting. Parents should take the lead at each meeting to briefly review the last conference and then set the stage for the current discussion. Likewise, at the end of the meeting, parents should summarize what has occurred and write this in the log. Many times the teacher will take this responsibility and give a photocopy to the parents, but parents are encouraged to take an active role if this process is not documented by another team member.

Table 12-2
PARENT DOCUMENTATION FORM

Date of Contact:

Team Member(s) Name(s) and Roles:

Purpose of Meeting:

Discussion:

Solutions Generated:

Solutions Decided Upon/Person Responsible for Implementation:

What Criteria Will Be Used to Judge Effectiveness of Intervention?

Next Meeting Date:

TYPICAL PARENT QUESTIONS/COMMENTS FOR SPECIAL EDUCATORS

It has been shocking to me that many professionals are unaware of public law pertaining to persons with disabilities. What can be done to raise awareness?

Although professionals working with students with and without special needs have a wealth of information, they need opportunities to become familiar with new techniques to help students, as well as new laws and regulations. Professionals and parents alike need access to this new information to help them provide optimal interdisciplinary services to students with special needs. By law and professional standards, all school personnel must have ongoing staff development every year. Optimally, these in-service opportunities should follow from the needs of particular school teams. Ask your school team how in-service topics are decided upon and who is the resource person who supervises staff development.

Keeping current about changes in the laws and regulations concerning the education of students with special needs can be overwhelming for everyone. IDEA mandates resources to help increase awareness of these issues. The reauthorization of IDEA in 1997 included significant changes in many areas regarding this concern. For the first time, significant resources have been authorized for in-service training for both parents and professionals. Information clearinghouses, regional resource centers, media and captioning services, and technology applications are available within each state to assist professionals and parents in raising awareness about disabilities.

Once again, parents need to take a proactive role in making sure that these resources are allocated for specific needs at the local level. For example, school professionals tell a family that they have never had a student with Tourette Syndrome before. An appropriate response from parents could include the suggestion that an in-service be conducted for the entire school staff by a knowledgeable person. The parents of the student with Tourette could offer to assist in the presentation of this in-service, perhaps focusing on how Tourette affects children outside of school, specifically at home and in the community. A panel of parents discussing children with this specific disability could offer interventions that have been successful. Parents could also help find resources for the school.

Often professionals who are unaware of a specific disability operate from a sense of fear of the unknown. Having an opportunity to learn more specific information as well as demystifying incorrect perceptions (e.g., "All students with Tourette use bad language and totally disrupt the general education class routine.") can benefit all team members.

The bottom line is this—money for professional development is embedded in the law. Find out how you can become a part of planning and delivering new information to your child's interdisciplinary team. Don't passively assume that your child's needs will be addressed in staff development activities. Remember, education goes two ways. You may often be called upon to be the educators of the educators. This can be done in a collaborative manner where all parties benefit from this new information, especially the student.

Dr. Schulz's Response:
The lack of professional knowledge of IDEA has also been surprising to me. For example, when I was teaching in a public school after the implementation of P.L. 94-142, I talked with my principal about a child who had severe behavior disorders. He stated, "Well, if he doesn't straighten up, we'll just send him home."

I agree with the author that parents should be more proactive in sharing their own knowledge. If parents are team members, it follows that it behooves them to share information with other team members. Many parents have become experts in the nature and characteristics of their child's disability and can be active in in-service training as well as informal conversations with professionals.

When I went back to school after having my children, I was in awe of my professors. One morning, I left my son, Billy, at school (he was in a special class) and went to my own class on communication disorders. The professor stated emphatically, "There are no girls with Mongolism [Down syndrome]." I was too intimidated to tell him that I had just left a room where three such girls were enrolled. Needless to say, I have gained confidence since that time and would now hasten to correct him.

How can a parent be a part of the education of peers of their child with mental retardation? I feel the need to help others (my child's peers) see my son as I see him.

Children with special needs often have difficulty with peer relations. Every child deserves to have a friend and to be a friend. Both teachers and parents can play a vital role in encouraging positive peer relationships. One way in which to accomplish this is through education about the disability; this dispels myths and presents the student as being more like others than different. Focusing on sameness rather than differences will facilitate acceptance.

Students often can be a resource in sharing information about their specific disability. A short teaching focus planned by the parent, student and teacher would be a good beginning to help raise awareness. This could be done formally as a structured part of the school day or informally in naturally occurring settings (e.g., lunchroom, playground, after-school care, school clubs, etc.). Additionally, inviting a sibling of a special needs student to the classroom may provide an opportunity for modeling of appropriate peer interactions.

Parents can play a vital role in this type of activity by supporting the school staff and perhaps being present during the discussion with the child's classmates. Parents could pull together a portfolio of photographs and memorabilia (awards from Special Olympics, artwork, notes form teachers and peers) showing their child participating in normally occurring childhood activities. This can help move the focus from the differences of the child with special needs to more emphasis on similarities.

Dr. Schulz's Response:

Research indicates that interaction among students with and without disabilities usually does not occur spontaneously in integrated classrooms. Interventions are needed to focus on facilitating such interaction. One approach is to teach communication skills directly to the child with disabilities; another approach is to teach peers to initiate and sustain communicative interaction with the child who has disabilities (Schulz & Carpenter, 1995). Both approaches require parent and teacher collaboration.

Peer tutoring is another way to bring students with and without disabilities together to accomplish defined goals. Helping relationships often turn into friendships. In one class for children with severe disabilities, the teacher instituted a peer tutoring program in collaboration with parents and other teachers. The peer tutors became so interested in the children with disabilities that they maintained their relationships throughout the summer and holidays.

This is another opportunity for parents to make suggestions and to work with other team members to initiate change.

CASE EXAMPLE

Tom is a fifth grader who has been experiencing difficulty with mathematics for several years. His parents have shared their concerns with his teacher and have expressed their frustration that Tom continues to struggle. They ask the classroom teacher what services are available for students like Tom who need more help than is typically provided in the general education classroom. The teacher tells Tom's parents about the Teacher Assistance Team that meets weekly and is composed of special education professionals and veteran general classroom teachers. Tom's teacher schedules him to be discussed at this forum the next week. She presents Tom's academic concerns to the Teacher Assistance Team. The other members of the team ask for specific information about Tom's performance both on standardized testing as well as more informal curriculum-based assessment. They ask Tom's teacher to bring this information to the next meeting to help the members develop a plan of action.

At the next meeting Tom's teacher shares the information. Although his current grade placement is 5.5, his standardized scores show him to be performing more like a third grader as shown by his grade equivalence score of 3.2. Tom's teacher also brings a considerable amount of daily work products showing that Tom does not have the skills for success in the fifth grade mathematics curriculum. The team recommends that a teacher's aide help Tom with some of the prerequisite skills needed for success in the classroom. The team decides on three remedial areas and gives curricular materials to the classroom teacher. They ask the teacher to report back to the team in three weeks after keeping daily data about Tom's performance.

After three weeks, the team reconvenes to talk about the impact of the first set of interventions. They ask Tom's parents to attend this meeting. His parents are interested in hearing what the Teacher Assistance Team will recommend to help their son academically, but they also raise the concern about how the many years of school failure have impacted his self-esteem. They ask about counseling services as well as remedial help for his academic delays.

The daily data collected over three weeks show minimal gains indicating a need for further evaluation by the special education team. The team, along with Tom's parents, recommends a comprehensive special education evaluation to assess his cognitive, academic, and social/emotional strengths and concerns. They put this in writing to the school principal and the school psychologist. This letter begins the process of having Tom formally evaluated for possible special education services.

Tom is evaluated by the school psychologist, the learning specialist, and the social worker. The learning specialist has a conference with Tom's classroom teacher to elicit more information about his learning style. She decides to visit the classroom and observe Tom doing a variety of classroom activities, including a large group activity, small group work, and independent seat work. The learning specialist uses an observation checklist form that has been created to document various behaviors of Tom, his teacher, and the classroom environment. The learning specialist schedules with the classroom teacher to visit three different times during mathematics instruction. After the third visit, she sits down with the teacher to discuss whether the behaviors observed were typical of Tom or, for some reason, were atypical. The psychologist and the social worker also interview the classroom teacher as part of their evaluations.

Although the psychologist, the learning specialist, and the social worker all have important information to share with the team when testing is complete, the classroom teacher remains a key source of team information. The classroom teacher has more opportunities to observe Tom on a daily basis than any of the other team members. Her insights will be considered carefully during the final discussion of the assessment findings.

At the team meeting, the team unanimously agrees that Tom is showing significant delays in his acquisition of mathematics abilities. They also determine that he qualifies for learning disabilities services in the area of mathematics and will begin receiving an hour of special help each day. Some of this help will be in the resource room staffed by the learning specialist, but most of it will be delivered in the general education classroom. Consultative services will also be given to the general education teacher on a weekly basis to give her support and ideas on how to help Tom throughout the day.

This consultative collaboration shows the important role educators play in helping students with special needs. Although other members of the assessment team may have more specific information about students with disabilities and how to help them, the general education teacher will be the one person who will continue to facilitate most of Tom's learning in the classroom. It is important that the classroom teacher and the special education teacher have ongoing communication regarding Tom's needs.

His parents will be contacted on a regular basis to update them about Tom's performance at school. It is possible that there will be a need to change his individual education plan if there is only limited success. Tom's teachers and parents will continue to have frequent communication with the understanding that any of the team members can ask for a revision of the IEP or another set of comprehensive assessment data. By keeping the focus on Tom's needs, the team can continue to work together to meet any future challenges.

Educators are an integral part of both the diagnostic and the intervention phases of working with students with special needs. Parents may often have multiple educators with whom to collaborate. Parents are encouraged to take an active part in coordinating efforts among educators and other team members to ensure that their child is receiving not just an appropriate education, as required by law, but an education that is carefully integrated and meets his or her multiple needs. A caring and effective teacher can make all the difference for both the child and the family. However, even the most effective teacher needs parent support and ideas in coming together to create an appropriate education for each child.

Editors' Note:

Colson and Carr provide a clear overview of IDEA and a useful review of its impact on special educators' roles and responsibilities. It is important that all team members (including parents) be current with respect to IDEA and other public laws. Such currency is critical to effective service delivery within and beyond the public school setting.

REFERENCES

Schulz, J. B., & Carpenter, C. D. (1995). *Mainstreaming exceptional students* (4th ed.). Boston: Allyn and Bacon.

Turnbull, A., Turnbull, R., Shank, M., & Leal, D. (1999). *Exceptional Lives* (2nd ed.). Upper Saddle River, NJ: Merrill.

Chapter 13

PSYCHOLOGY

N. S. Vellet and M. Reese

MAJOR ROLES AND RESPONSIBILITIES PLAYED BY PSYCHOLOGY

Psychologists observe and examine the behavior of individuals in an effort to understand how we think, learn and develop, perceive, feel, act, interact with others, and understand ourselves. Psychology shares this focus on human behavior with other disciplines, such as speech and language pathology and special education. Actually, there is considerable overlap among fields in the behaviors studied and methods used. Nonetheless, the various disciplines involved in conducting comprehensive and coordinated interdisciplinary services to children and adolescents offer different emphases, perspectives, and information. For example, the roles that psychology could play are numerous, including trying to answer questions about the individual's developmental competencies and strengths, emotional growth, behavior problems, the influence of the home environment on development, and the appropriateness of an educational placement. Even though the scope of work is great, the psychologist's major roles involve assessment, treatment, and consultation.

Assessment

A major responsibility of psychology is assessment. This could include assessing an individual's cognitive abilities (i.e., intelligence), daily living skills (i.e., adaptive behavior), social and emotional status, academic achievement, and family functioning. It could also include functional analyses of challenging behaviors. Assessment is typically completed through the use of standardized tests, which measure a specific aspect of behavior, feelings, self-perception, etc. These tests are given in a highly specific manner that enables each person taking the test to have an equal chance for success.

Some of the tests that psychologists give involve the parents or teachers rating the behavior of the individual. It is an advantage to have a number of ratings so that different perceptions can be taken into account, as well as behavioral differences in different environments. Test results are translated into numbers so that the child can be compared to other children who are the same age or are in the same grade. Criterion referenced tests may also be used to determine a child's progress on individualized objectives.

Treatment

In addition to assessment, psychologists are frequently involved in treatment. The treatment role of psychologists might involve assisting parents with managing an individual's behavior problems. Treatment might also include helping the individual with a disability to cope better in difficult social situations (social skills training). For example, the person with a disability may show interest in developing peer relationships but not know how to start a conversation. A person may also have difficulty accepting negative feedback from a teacher or giving negative feedback to peers. Additionally, treatment could include assisting the individual in coping with unusually intense emotions such as fear or anger. In many cases, the person with a disability can be taught how to monitor his or her own emotional state and to respond, if necessary, with calming, relaxation techniques. For example, the person may become very frightened when going to the school nurse. The psychologist may have the person imagine and/or role play going to the nurse while relaxing at the same time. The psychological treatment might also involve helping a person manage behaviors that are problematic through self-control techniques. Self-control teaches the person how to observe his or her own behavior, record whether the behavior occurred or not, evaluate the behavior, and give feedback to him or herself as to how he or she is doing. Self-control may be used to help eliminate undesirable habits such as overeating or nail biting. Self-control techniques can also be applied to behaviors that need to occur more often. For example, getting all homework assignments and needed books before leaving school, starting a conversation with peers, and completing all self-care skills in the morning may be targets for self-control programs.

Consultation

In addition to treatment, a psychologist may take on the role of a consultant. The consultation request could be very broad such as how to structure an integrated classroom. The consultation could also be very narrow. For example, the psychologist might be asked to observe a student who is having difficulty in learning a particular educational objective and to suggest alternative teaching strategies. Psychologists are frequently asked to consult on behavioral difficulties. There may be an entire classroom that is particularly disruptive or one individual with a challenging behavior who may be interfering with all the students' learning. The first step in behavioral consultation is to look at any environmental or medical condition that might be contributing to the problem. For example, a classroom without air conditioning on a warm spring day might be particularly prone to producing challenging behaviors. Similarly, a student with an undiagnosed ear infection might have a great deal of difficulty when concentration is required in class.

A second step in behavioral consultation might be setting up an incentive system for the class or the individual who is exhibiting behavioral difficulties. For example, the class might be divided into teams and the team with the fewest disruptions may get extra recess time. For an individual, a home note system might be set up. If the student exhibits fewer than two disruptions, parents might mark the calendar. When there are a specific number of marks on the calendar, the student might get a special trip.

CONTRIBUTIONS OF PSYCHOLOGY TO INTERDISCIPLINARY PRACTICE

Psychologist's Role in Assessment

One of the primary interdisciplinary roles of psychologists is to provide assessment data. Psychologists can provide various types of assessment data to the interdisciplinary team. As noted above, assessment can be applied to cognitive abilities, daily living skills, social and emotional status, academic achievement, family functioning, etc. It would be instructive, at this point, to define assessment terms, outline some common procedures, and explain why a particular assessment might be important to the interdisciplinary team.

Definitions

There are probably as many definitions of intelligence as there are researchers and theoreticians studying the topic. The common themes that run through the definitions of intelligence proposed by many psychologists are (1) the capacity to learn from experience, (2) the ability to adapt to the environment, (3) the ability to understand and control one's thinking processes (such as during problem-solving, reasoning, and decision-making), and (4) the variance of intelligence from culture to culture (Sattler, 1992). Considerable research shows that many factors interact to influence the course of mental development, including the genes the child inherits from his or her parents, maturational issues (e.g., complications of labor and delivery, childhood illnesses, malnutrition), and home environmental variables (e.g., emphasis placed on achievement motivation, encouragement of language development) (Sattler, 1992).

There are many reasons for including a measure of intelligence as part of an interdisciplinary assessment (Lincoln, Kaufman, & Kaufman, 1995). For example, several specific diagnoses require that a standardized measure of general ability or intelligence be administered, including mental retardation and specific learning disabilities (American Psychiatric Association, 1994). Level of intelligence is strongly associated with one's adaptive capabilities and potential. In addition, intelligence is an integral aspect of one's personality structure (Lincoln, Kaufman, & Kaufman, 1995). One of the final reasons for including an assessment of intelligence in an interdisciplinary evaluation is that it provides a sample of the child's behavior in a fairly systematic manner (Lincoln, Kaufman, & Kaufman, 1995).

Adaptive behavior reflects a person's competence in functioning and maintaining oneself independently (e.g., independently caring for one's toileting and hygiene needs) and in meeting the social demands of one's environment (e.g., knowing how to initiate and end a conversation) (Sattler, 1992). Definitions of adaptive behavior are rather imprecise, as it is not possible to know the environmental conditions in which an individual is required to function. In addition, the adaptive behaviors that are most relevant to an individual will vary depending on one's stage of development. For example, increasing independence around toileting issues is an important aspect of adaptive functioning during the preschool years, whereas social and economic independence become particularly salient beginning in early adulthood (Sattler, 1992). An evaluation of adaptive functioning is important in the team process. For example, strengths and weaknesses may be taken into account in identifying educational goals and objectives. Also, standardized test results from various disciplines that are obtained in a one-on-one testing situation might be compared to adaptive functioning in corresponding areas.

In an effort to understand a child's social and emotional functioning, a psychologist could explore the child's sense of self, capacity for self-regulation, emotional factors (e.g., anxiety, depression, motivation), adjustment in regard to school and home, attachment to caregivers, peer relations (e.g., social skills, status, and maturity), and family functioning. Assessment of social and emotional functioning may be important for the interdisciplinary team in identifying appropriate services (e.g., counseling or resource room) or identifying appropriate goals and objectives (e.g., social skills, self-control).

Academic achievement refers to learning a child acquires from the school and home environments. Preacademic skills (e.g., attentional skills, language processing, auditory comprehension) as well as academic ability (e.g., performance in reading, spelling, and arithmetic) are important aspects of academic achievement. Academic achievement is important to the team in identifying specific learning disabilities and/or devising educational strategies and/or appropriate goals and objectives for the educational plan.

The definition of family functioning is complex, including such factors as family structure, the roles family members fill within the family, the quality of family relationships, parenting styles, parental mental health, and the communication patterns within the family system. Family stress and ability to adjust to and cope with challenges (e.g., to the changing developmental needs of children), the support of the extended family, the commitment of family members to solving family problems, and the family's problem-solving style are also important aspects of family functioning. Family functioning is important to the team in determining family strengths. Family strengths and needs may impact the family's ability to carry out educational strategies in the home.

The focus of conducting a functional analysis of challenging behavior is two-part. The first part of a functional analysis is to identify the environmental conditions in which problem behaviors such as aggression, destruction, and self-injury occur. Environment in this context is broadly defined. Environment can include the external environment, as well as the internal physiological environment. When conducting a functional analysis, it is important to note whether the problem behaviors occur more frequently in conditions such as crowds, noise, high temperature, lack of leisure materials, group instruction, etc. Physiological environmental conditions may include pain, illness, allergies, menses, medication changes, or side effects, etc. The second part of a functional analysis is to determine the purpose or function the behavior is serving for the individual. Some problem behavior such as aggression or self-injury may occur in order to obtain attention. Other problem behaviors may occur as a result of difficult tasks. Still other problem behaviors, such as repetitive movements, may occur because of the sensory sensations the behavior produces. For example, hitting one's ear when there is an ear infection may temporarily relieve the pain. Sitting and rocking may produce a type of stimulation, called vestibular stimulation, which may be quite rewarding or reinforcing for the individual. The purpose of identifying the functions of problem behaviors is that many behaviors have a communicative purpose. If the communicative function can be identified, teachers and parents may teach a more appropriate behavior that would assist the person in meeting his or her needs. The functional analysis is relevant to the team, in that the education environment or illness can be discussed. Also, replacement skills that have a communicative or sensory function can be targeted as educational objectives.

Common Measurement Tools

Perhaps the leading intelligence tests are those developed by David Wechsler. There are two designed for children: the Wechsler Intelligence Scale for Children-Third Edition (WISC-III; Wechsler, 1991), which is intended for children six years to 17 years, and the Wechsler Preschool and Primary Scale of Intelligence-Revised (WPPSI-R; Wechsler, 1989), which is intended for children ranging in age from three to seven years. Both tests focus on measuring skills that are considered relevant to successful functioning in school. In addition, both the WISC-III and WPPSI-R are divided into a verbal scale (which includes tasks measuring verbal comprehension and expression) and a performance scale (which includes tasks measuring visual analysis, visual-motor integration, and motor speed). The tests, therefore, yield both an overall intelligence quotient (IQ) and separate verbal and performance IQs.

Some individuals score about evenly on both the verbal and performance scales while others score higher on one group of subtests than the other. Actually, it is possible to find evidence of uneven organization of cognitive abilities when there is a significant discrepancy between the individual's performance on the verbal and performance subtests. For example, it has been found that individuals with receptive language disorders have significantly lower Verbal IQ scores compared to their Performance IQ scores (Lincoln, Kaufman, & Kaufman, 1995).

The Kaufman Assessment Battery for Children (K-ABC; Kaufman & Kaufman, 1983) was designed to assess the intelligence and achievement of 2 1/2- to 12 1/2-year-old children. The Mental Processing scales of the K-ABC measure the child's ability to solve problems sequentially (i.e., solving problems in which the information is presented in a sequence) and simultaneously (i.e., integrating many pieces of information to solve problems), with an emphasis on the process used to produce correct solutions. The K-ABC also includes an Achievement Scale, which measures a child's knowledge of facts, language concepts, and school-related skills. A special nonverbal scale, made up of those subtests that may be administered in pantomime and responded to motorically, is also provided to assess the mental processing of hearing-impaired, speech- and language-impaired, and non-English speaking children ages four through 12 1/2.

The Bayley Scales of Infant Development-Second Edition (BSID-II; Bayley, 1993) constitute one of the most widely used instruments for evaluating the developmental status of children from one to 42 months. The BSID-II consist of three components: the Mental Scale (assessing perceptual, memory, problem-solving, and communication), the Motor Scale (intended to measure control of the body, muscular coordination, and manipulation skills), and the Infant Behavior Record (used to evaluate the child's emotional and behavioral responses to the examiner and testing environment).

Some children have characteristics (e.g., difficulties around establishing social relationships, poor communication skills, unusual responses to sensory stimuli) that may create challenges in the testing situation. For example, some children may show little or no interest in the tasks or in interacting with the psychologist and typical methods of providing encouragement (e.g., smiling) may be of limited effectiveness. Under these circumstances, the psychologist should use testing procedures and measures that are appropriate and geared to the child's strengths and limitations. For example, depending on the child's characteristics, the psychologist may need to adjust the speed and complexity of his or her speech, the amount of praise and encouragement provided, and the amount of redirection given. Moreover, when working with some children psychologists may need to utilize instruments that measure cognitive abilities by means of nonverbal items (e.g., Leiter International Performance Scale, Leiter, 1948; PEP-R, Schopler & Reichler, 1979).

The Vineland Adaptive Behavior Scales (VABS) (Sparrow, Balla, & Cicchetti, 1984) is one of the most widely used tools for the assessment of adaptive behavior. The VABS assesses the ability to perform daily activities required for personal and social sufficiency in individuals ranging in age from birth through 19 years. The VABS is typically completed by a trained examiner through interviewing a respondent familiar with the behavior of the child in question (i.e., parent or teacher). Adaptive behavior is measured in four domains: Communication (receptive, expressive, written), Daily Living Skills (personal living habits, domestic task performance, behavior in the community), Socialization (interaction with others, including play, use of free time), and Motor Skills (gross and fine motor coordination). These four domains are combined to form the Adaptive Behavior Composite. The VABS also contains a Maladaptive Behavior domain to assess undesirable behaviors that may interfere with the child's adaptive behavior (Sattler, 1992).

The social and emotional problems that some children experience can be complex and demand an assessment to determine the primary difficulty that requires some intervention. It is important to remember that seeking help for a child is usually prompted by the dissatisfaction of adults (usually the parents or school personnel) with the child's behavior at school, home, or peer relations. Given that the parents are the ones bringing the child in for evaluation, it is possible that the child perceives the situation very differently (e.g., does not think that a problem exists or has explanations for it). Therefore, the psychologist should conduct an interview with the child and parent(s) to obtain background information concerning the child's development, prior adjustment, and current adjustment. Parenting behaviors and methods also may be explored. Moreover, direct observation, self-report questionnaires, behavior checklist, and projective techniques (e.g., drawings, projective story telling) can also be used to assess the social and emotional functioning of children and adolescents. Psychologists assess children and adolescents with a wide range of adjustment difficulties, including conduct problems, brain injury, depression, fears, anxieties, and social relationship problems. Examples of commonly used measures of social and emotional functioning of children are the parent-completed Child Behavior Checklist 4-18 (Achenbach, 1991), the Youth Self-Report 11-18 (Achenbach, 1991), the Revised Children's Manifest Anxiety Scale (Reynolds & Richmond, 1985), the Child Depression Inventory (Kovacs, 1982), Self-Perception Profile for Children (Harter, 1985), and the Roberts Apperception Test (McArthur & Roberts, 1982).

Common achievement tests include the Wide Range Achievement Test-Third Edition (Jastak, 1993) that contains reading, spelling, and arithmetic subtests. Similarly, the Kaufman Test of Educational Achievement (Kaufman & Kaufman, 1985) contains subtests assessing reading decoding and comprehension, spelling, and arithmetic applications and computation. The Woodcock-Johnson Psycho-Educational Battery (Woodcock, 1977) evaluates functioning in three areas: cognitive, achievement, and interest. Furthermore, the examiner should carefully observe all aspects of the child's test performance, including what types of errors the child made and the response style used.

It has been argued that the family context has a pervasive, continuous, and personal influence on the development of its members (Carlson, 1990). A variety of methods have been utilized to evaluate family functioning, including self-report questionnaires, interviews, formal and informal observations, behavior ratings, projective measures, and structured tasks. Moreover, in an assessment of family context, many areas could be examined, including family rules about how to relate to one another, family resources, priorities, and concerns, family developmental stage (e.g., a family with young children vs. a family with adolescents), family stress and coping, the family's subjective reality (e.g., the discrepancy between behaviors and perceptions), and the presenting problem of the child or adolescent as possibly a sign of a systemic problem. In addition, it may be useful to explore the parent-child, marital, and siblings' relationships. Commonly used measures of family functioning include the Family Adaptability, Cohesion, and Expressiveness Scale (Olson, Portner, & Lavee, 1985), the Family Environment Scale (Moos & Moos, 1986), and the Family Relations Test (Bene, 1985).

There are a number of methods to collect functional analysis data. The simplest method is to conduct an interview. The purpose of the interview is to obtain information regarding the type of problem behaviors that are being seen, the external environmental, and physiological conditions that seem to result in the problem behaviors, and the purpose or function of the behaviors. At times, the behavioral interview is all that is possible, but hopefully the behavioral interview may lead to a more direct observational approach to conducting the functional analysis. Bailey and Pyles (1989) and O'Neill, Horner, Albin, Storey, and Sprague (1990) have provided an interview format for those conducting a functional analysis. These interviews contain such items as whether there are medical conditions that seem to relate to the problem behaviors, whether the behaviors occur more often or less often at particular times of the day, in particular settings or with specific people or tasks. The interview also asks the parent to judge the function or purpose of the problem behaviors.

Another method of conducting a functional analysis is to use rating scales, checklists, and questionnaires. For example, answers to a 16-question motivational assessment scale (Durand & Crimmins, 1988) can provide information about the potential functions that are maintaining the problem behavior. The functions this instrument assesses include obtaining attention, obtaining designed objects or events, avoiding tasks, avoiding demands, and either avoiding or obtaining sensory input.

As noted above, however, the best way of conducting a functional analysis is through direct observations; parents and teachers are often asked to help with these observations. O'Neill et al. (1990) developed one of the most sophisticated direct observation techniques available. The data sheet involves a matrix in which episodes of the target behavior are recorded. The data sheet provides information as to time of day and specific physiological environmental conditions that are in effect at the time of the problem behavior. The matrix also asks observers to judge the function or purpose of the problem behavior at the time the behavior occurs. For example, parents and teachers are asked to judge whether the behavior appears to serve the purpose of recruiting attention, escaping from tasks, obtaining desirable events, or avoiding undesirable events, etc.

Psychologist's Role of Interpretation

The psychologist will also maintain close contact with the other team members throughout the course of the interdisciplinary process. The psychologist must explain the results of his or her evaluation to other team members and the child's parents. To this end, the psychologist may need to explain measurement concepts such as normal curve, standard scores, and percentiles.

Knowledge of measurement concepts will enable team members and parents to evaluate more effectively the psychometric properties of the tests being used during the assessment of their child or adolescent. In addition, knowledge of these concepts may enhance parents' understanding of their child.

In addition to explaining measurement concepts, the psychologist must be able to translate those concepts into how scores on a specific measurement device might impact every day functioning of the individual. The psychologist must be able to relate how psychological test results impact and relate to findings of other disciplines so that a cohesive picture of the child's strengths and needs can be described.

Psychologist's Role in Treatment Collaboration

Once the interdisciplinary assessment phase has been completed and strengths and needs have been identified by the team, this information should be translated into an action plan. The role of the psychologist is to help identify how psychological evaluation results might be translated into important goals and objectives. For example, needs from the adaptive behavior assessment can frequently be translated into functional skills. The psychologist must also collaborate with other team members in terms of how psychological findings might impact on learning objectives carried out in the classroom, speech therapy, or at home. For example, a child with attentional difficulties might learn faster with short, frequent opportunities to practice.

THE ROLES PARENTS TYPICALLY PLAY IN THE OPTIMAL INTERDISCIPLINARY SERVICE PROVISION OF PSYCHOLOGY

Interdisciplinary process includes at least six phases: (1) referral and preinterview data gathering, (2) parent interview, (3) assessment and observation, (4) integration and synthesis of information, (5) sharing findings and writing reports, and (6) treatment implementation. An optimal interdisciplinary service should involve collaboration between the professionals and the parents in understanding the child and family during each of these phases. For example, during the parent interview, the psychologist should communicate to the parents or other primary caregivers that they are partners in the evaluation process, to which they will be making a distinct contribution. Parents should be given the opportunity to share their perceptions of the child's strengths, difficulties, and needs and should discuss the issues to be explored in the assessment. Moreover, families should be encouraged to be the primary decision-makers throughout the assessment process and must be supported in this regard. All of the members of the interdisciplinary team must recognize and respect the fact that cultures vary in beliefs, values, and traditions concerning family roles and relationships, child-rearing techniques, communication, view of disability, and styles of interaction, particularly in relation to members of the helping professions (Erikson, 1997; Dunst, Trivette, & Deal, 1994; Reichard, 1997). In addition, the professionals must recognize that partnerships encompass families, interdisciplinary teams, and community members from many agencies.

While the psychologist is asking interview questions or having the parents fill out behavior checklists, parents must give frank, objective information. If parents do not understand a question, they must feel free to ask for clarification. Sometimes the psychologist will ask the parent to collect information as to how the child is behaving at home or in other environments. Parents should give the psychologist information as to the best ways of collecting the needed information. For example, a psychologist conducting a functional analysis of a particular behavior problem might ask the parent to write down what happened before the incident, how long the incident lasted, and what the parent did. This information can be time-consuming to obtain, particularly with problems that occur frequently. If the parent does not have time to record the information, an inaccurate picture of the problem might be obtained. The parent and the psychologist need to collaborate on how to get accurate information.

Another role of the parent is to help with education. Before and during the evaluation of the child, the parents can give information as to how to get the child's best performance. Parents can also provide information as to subtle cues that the child is becoming tired. Parents should give the psychologist some impression of how the child performed and whether his or her performance was typical.

Parents have an important role when assessment results are being discussed. Parents should be encouraged to ask questions and make comments. It is important that parents understand what the evaluation means and what recommendations are being made. During the interpretive meeting (when the results of the evaluation and recommendations are discussed with the parents), feedback should be elicited from the parents regarding their perception of the needs of the child. In addition, information about existing community services and supports the parents feel comfortable accessing should also be obtained.

Another parent role is to assist with treatment. As psychological treatments are being implemented, parents need to provide the psychologist with feedback as to the impact on the child's life. As with assessment of problem behaviors, treatment data might require the parents to record occurrences of the problem behaviors. How these data are collected can be very time-consuming and the process can be streamlined with good collaboration efforts between the psychologist and the parents. Also, the manner in which treatments are implemented will require a great deal of parent input. Parents frequently are responsible for carrying out support plans that assist individuals who display challenging behaviors. Parents know their child best and can identify the best way of implementing parts of support plans so that plans work and the impact on other activities a family must carry out is minimized. Parents also can give insight as to how treatment is impacting various family members and the whole family system.

Finally, parents have a role in giving the psychologist feedback about services. Parents should be asked to complete a questionnaire so that feedback can be obtained about their perceptions of the entire process. For example, parents could be asked to rate the importance of, and their satisfaction regarding, various issues including the team's ability to (1) listen to their description of their child, (2) explain their child's difficulties, (3) answer their questions, and (4) be sensitive to their cultural background.

TYPICAL PARENT QUESTIONS/COMMENTS FOR PSYCHOLOGY

I am still puzzled and resentful. I desperately continue to search for the cause of my child's autism. I had amniocentesis at 17 weeks and results were normal. I just had genetic testing, and the results were also normal. What causes this?

We do not know the cause of autism and there are probably several causes. In fact, many have indicated there is probably more than one type of autism. What we do know is that autism is a neurobiological disorder. There are a number of biological causes; however, none of them are unique to autism. Some prenatal factors include intrauterine rubella, tuberous sclerosis, and chromosomal disorders such as Fragile X. Perinatal difficulties during birth probably have little role in autism. Postnatal conditions that may be associated with autism are untreated phenylketonuria and herpes simplex encephalitis. Known causes for autism have varied in the literature from 10 percent to 30 percent.

Recent evidence suggests that genetics is very important in those types of autism in which there are no associated neurological conditions. For example, there is a 3 percent to 8 percent risk of recurrence in families with one affected child. So far, no specific gene for autism has been identified, although a possible link to serotonin transport gene has been suggested. Serotonin is a neurotransmitter that helps the brain transmit messages from one nerve cell to the next.

Recent research has also examined what areas of the brain might be involved in autism. Again, there is neither a coherent anatomical or biological diagnostic test that has been developed. Preliminary findings have found that there may be a lack of a certain type of cell in the cerebral cortex. The cerebral cortex is the switchboard of the brain, which controls sensory input signals, as well as controlling movement. Routine brain imaging, however, has usually not revealed anything primary to autism.

What kinds of things are being done to treat aggressive behavior in children with developmental disabilities? It is tough when my son tries to hit me or hurt me because he is frustrated. I don't like being afraid of my child.

Behavioral approaches, at times combined with medication, are the most effective means of treating aggressive behavior in children with developmental disabilities. The old thinking, in terms of behavioral techniques, assumed that we needed to find the right consequences for aggressive behavior. Newer thinking is that we need to conduct a functional analysis of aggressive behavior. Aggressive behavior may be caused by certain environmental conditions such as crowds and overstimulation, the lack of leisure materials, pain, and illness. Aggressive behavior may also serve a variety of functions. In some individuals, the aggression may serve to recruit or maintain an interaction with important people. In other situations, the aggressive behavior may serve to avoid or escape from demand situations. In still other situations, the behavior may result from avoiding undesirable activities or events. Treatment protocols cannot be established without conducting a functional analysis that can be used to modify the environment and teach appropriate replacement skills.

Some of the newer techniques that have been researched are described below. For example, if aggressive behavior occurs to maintain an interaction, a picture book or a remnant book can be used by individuals with developmental disabilities to maintain attention after they have appropriately gotten someone to pay attention to them. For aggressive behavior that occurs to escape instructions, it is sometimes desirable to give children instructions in which there is a high likelihood that they will comply prior to giving an instruction in which there is low probability of compliance. This technique is like warming the child up and establishing rapport prior to giving the child a demand in which there is high likelihood of aggressive behavior. For children who exhibit aggressive behavior to escape or avoid undesirable events, it is often useful to establish a picture system for these children. A picture system represents the activities that are going to occur during the day. This gives the child some forewarning of what events are going to occur. This may be very beneficial if the child has poor understanding of language and instructions. The picture schedule can be arranged so that less desirable activities or events are always followed by highly desirable or reinforcing activities. The child can be shown that if he/she can get through a task that is not desirable, then he/she will be able to go out and do something that is really fun. Another advantage of the picture schedule is that it takes the pressure off of parents to constantly give children directions as to what to do. The picture schedule essentially tells them what to do. At times, giving the child choices with respect to how their daily activities are going to be carried out can also be beneficial when children escape or avoid particular activities or events.

Medications may be necessary for the treatment of aggressive behavior. Medications may be of assistance if the child seems to explode, and there are no particular environmental conditions setting the occasion for the behavior. Medications may also be of assistance if the child has rituals that they have to adhere to, and redirecting the child from these rituals sets the occasion for aggressive behavior. Additionally, medications may be useful when a child has difficulty attending for long periods of time and is very distractible. Attention to task can be very demanding when a child has a short attention span.

A final point is that it is very beneficial to try to figure out what the child is trying to communicate through aggressive behavior, and to teach the child a more appropriate way of manipulating his or her environment.

How should I discipline my young child with mental retardation?

Frequently, when people hear the word "discipline," they think of consequences for inappropriate behavior. Usually these consequences are ways of punishing inappropriate behavior, and may include mild consequences such as briefly removing the child from the situation to more severe consequences such as spanking the child. Discipline should be thought of as teaching. There are two parts to teaching. The first part is whether the child actually knows how to behave in a particular situation. Children exhibit inappropriate behavior simply because they do not know how to behave. The second part is whether the child is motivated to behave appropriately in certain situations when he or she has the skills. Some children may find it much easier and a lot more rewarding to behave inappropriately even when they have appropriate skills.

Given that discipline is an educational task, there are important rules for the parent. Parents should have rules as to what they expect of children. These rules should be very concrete. There should be explicit consequences, particularly for behaving appropriately in situations. There should be forewarning of what will happen if the child behaves inappropriately. Much of the concentration in terms of discipline techniques should be on teaching appropriate skills, and catching the child being good. Catching the child behaving appropriately might include the use of priming. Priming is a technique in which parents forewarn the child as to appropriate behavior in a particular problematic situation. For example, many children have difficulty being ignored when their parents are on the telephone. Parents might discuss ahead of time that when the telephone rings, parents will direct the child's attention toward an appropriate activity. If the child is able to occupy his or her time during the telephone conversation, then special rewards will be provided.

Can you give me suggestions on how to deal with changes associated with adolescence? I have a son with a disability who has no understanding why certain things are happening to him.

Adolescence is a time in which there are a number of hormonal changes. These changes can be reflected in a number of emotional states, which may be difficult to understand for an adolescent with a disability. For those adolescents who can self-monitor emotional states, it is a matter of teaching the individual how to determine his or her own feelings and to act appropriately on those emotions. Programs can be set up to teach an individual how to self-record emotional feelings. This can be translated into simplistic terms such as circling drawings of faces that reflect different emotional states. The individual then can be taught how to react to those emotional states in appropriate ways. There are some adolescents, however, with significant disabilities who may not have the language skills in order to teach them to self-monitor. This makes the situation somewhat more difficult. In this situation, emotional states may interact with environmental situations to create a number of problematic behaviors. For example, the individual may be in a very agitated mood for no explicable reason. While in this mood, environmental situations such as crowds and/or difficult tasks can create problems such as aggression or self-injurious behavior. In this situation, it is important to teach the individuals in the person's life how to recognize emotional states. For example, there may be subtle changes in facial expression. It is also important to identify what environmental conditions may interact with these emotional states to create problematic behaviors. A possible strategy when individuals in the person's environment recognize emotional states that may precipitate problematic behavior is redirection to environments that don't interact with those states. For example, we once worked with an individual who, upon entering adolescence, had unexplained bouts of agitation. During these agitated states, the individual would frown and grimace. If the person was in noisy, crowded environments and given a number of instructions when he was in this agitated state, it often resulted in self-injurious behavior. We taught individuals working with this person to recognize agitation, place the individual in a quiet, less crowded environment, and minimize demands. This frequently produced a de-escalation of agitation and permitted programming to resume much quicker than ignoring the agitated facial expression and allowed continuation of with general routines.

Dr. Schulz's Response:

Adolescence is difficult for all children. Add to this the frustration of being different, of having a difficult time in school, and one wonders how children with disabilities and their parents survive. At an age when different shoes are life-threatening, having a strange looking body or face is indeed frustrating. I remember seeing a film about a boy with Down syndrome who said to his mother, "I hate the way I look." This prompted me to ask Billy, "How do you feel about the way you look?" He responded immediately, "I'm a handsome man!" I don't know where that confidence came from (because it is true) but I know there are many areas in which he feels terribly insecure. The family, as always, is so important in helping the child see his or her strengths. It is also important to attend to the appropriateness of clothing and grooming.

Another observation of mine is that adolescence may come late, and some of the behaviors we see in adulthood may illustrate this fact. Mood swings, irritability, and seclusion may develop at a later time. Understanding that this may be adolescence is helpful.

I found that there is resistance to working on my child's social skills. Should this be a viable target of treatment?

Social skills are probably one of the most important targets for individuals with disabilities. Displaying appropriate skills in social situations can greatly enhance quality of life. For example, a person with good social skills is more likely to be integrated in a variety of community settings. Individuals with good social skills are also more likely to be able to establish friendships, which may be life-long. There is documented evidence that when it comes to employment, social skills are more important than being able to carry out job routines with respect to continued employment. Social skills training is an area that falls within a number of interdisciplinary professions. For example, social workers often run social skills training groups. The groups can also be conducted by psychologists. Additionally, speech and language pathologists working on pragmatics may be involved with social skills training. It is important when conducting social skills training, however, that individuals be given opportunities to practice throughout the day. Although an individual has a skill within a defined training setting, it does not ensure the skill would generalize or will occur in other environments. All individuals in the person's life should be able to recognize opportunities for appropriate social skills, prime the individual in terms of appropriate social behaviors, and then be available to reinforce appropriate social skills as they occur. This requires a great deal of team collaboration in that everybody knows the problem social areas, can prompt the appropriate skills and provide the individual with feedback.

Dr. Schulz's Response

Social skills, like language, develop in social settings. Inclusion of children with disabilities in all aspects of life contributes to the development of such skills. It is important for teachers and parents to realize that their children with disabilities may need preinclusion training, and that every transition (daycare to school, elementary to secondary school, school to adult living) requires advanced planning and training in social as well as academic and vocational areas. For example, some children may need to know the importance of smiling and greeting others, of shaking hands instead of hugging and listening as well as talking.

CASE EXAMPLE

Bob is a two-year, ten-month-old boy who was referred for an interdisciplinary evaluation. Bob's parents were very concerned about his slow development of language abilities, lack of eye contact, ability to interact with other children, and his preoccupation with certain parts of objects. Bob was also described as very particular about his routines. He prefers to play with his toy cars and line them up. Bob is very fascinated with looking in the windows of the cars.

Bob has been attending The Early Language Program where he has been working on expanding his understanding of language and his ability to express himself. Bob's teacher and speech therapist report that he is very independent and prefers to get things for himself rather than ask. He does have a few words but seldom uses them. Most of his words represent his favorite objects; however, even when he wants those objects, Bob seldom speaks. He usually takes his mom's or dad's hand and puts their hand on what he wants.

Bob's parents and the people working with him at school also report that he will become aggressive and at times bangs his head. These behaviors typically occur when his parents or teacher try to direct Bob's attention toward necessary activities of daily living such as toileting or to preacademic tasks. Aggression and self-injurious behaviors were very likely to occur when people tried to redirect his attention from his cars. The behaviors also occurred when Bob was having difficulty with a task and became frustrated.

Bob was seen by a psychologist as a part of an interdisciplinary evaluation in a transdisciplinary arena type of assessment. He had previously been seen by a developmental medicine team. Metabolic screens, as well as genetic testing, had ruled out any medical problems that may contribute to Bob's lack of communication and social difficulties. The assessments chosen by the psychologist included a nonverbal test of intelligence called the Leiter. This cognitive assessment was chosen because of Bob's difficulty with expressive language, and reported difficulty with understanding speech. The Psycho-Educational Profile-Revised was also administered. This assessment provided a profile of different developmental areas, and helped to identify skills that Bob already had in his repertoire, as well as skills that were emerging and might be emphasized at home and in educational settings. In order to get his parents' perspective of how he was doing in adaptive areas, the Vineland Adaptive Behavior Scale was conducted to provide a profile of communication, socialization, daily living, and motor skills. Since Bob did present with some characteristics of autism, the Childhood Autism Rating Scale was completed. This is an observational measure which rates various aspects of autism including relating to people, imitation, unusual body movements, unusual behaviors when presented with sensory stimuli, delayed or unusual language, etc.

Parents also reported that Bob did exhibit aggressive and self-injurious behavior. Because of these difficulties, the psychologist conducted a functional analysis interview to determine any physiological and environmental factors that might contribute to his behavior, as well as the potential purpose or functions of these behaviors. Bob was also seen in the arena assessment by a speech and language pathologist to look more closely at his understanding of language and his ability to express himself. Additionally, he was seen by an occupational therapist to assess any sensory qualities that may be contributing to his developmental delays, as well as appropriate and inappropriate behaviors.

During the assessment, it was noted that Bob showed awareness of the presence of the examiner but displayed very poor eye contact. Bob displayed no speech. He did use contact gestures in which he would take the examiner's hand and pull the examiner's hand toward an object to request objects. He also used contact gestures such as pushing the examiner's hand away in order to refuse test items. Bob did display interest in all objects presented to him. He had difficulty transitioning from one test item to the next. Bob preferred to manipulate objects as he saw fit, often organizing them and lining them up. When the examiner tried to give Bob more direct instructions as to what to do, he frequently would push the examiner's hand away. If instructions continued, Bob would become aggressive and exhibit self-injurious behavior that included slapping his face.

Bob's nonverbal cognitive abilities were measured in the low average range, although it was felt by the examiner and impressions confirmed by his parents, that Bob could have done better. His refusal of directions to complete tasks and his interest in lining up and organizing items probably contributed to somewhat lower scores than might represent his potential. Bob's profile on the Psycho-Educational Profile-Revised revealed extreme variability in skills. For example, imitation and his ability to understand and express himself using language was measured at about 12 months. Bob's ability to use his vision in order to match and integrate objects and to use a pencil to draw designs was a strength for him. These abilities were measured at closer to the three year level. Bob's scores on the Vineland Adaptive Behavior Scale also revealed a great deal of variability. Communication and socialization were weak areas for Bob. These abilities were measured at a little over one year. Motor skills were a strength for Bob. These skills were measured at closer to two years and six months. Daily living abilities were in-between these strengths and weaknesses, and were measured at about one year, nine months. Results from the Childhood Autism Rating Scale placed Bob into the moderate range of autism. Most affected areas included Bob's difficulty relating to people, his poor imitation abilities, and difficulty with understanding and using language. Less affected areas included unusual body movements, abnormal sensory processing, and unusual activity level. Bob's ability to adapt to change was moderately affected, and he displayed moderately unusual emotional responses in that once he began a tantrum, he had difficulty calming down.

Results from the speech and language evaluation also supported the difficulties with expressive and receptive language abilities. Bob used contact gestures or holding a person's hand in order to communicate. He communicated at a very low rate. Much of his communication was to request desired objects, or to protest. It was also felt by the speech and language pathologist that much of the tantrum behavior had a communicative function in that Bob was protesting undesirable and/or difficult tasks. Results from the occupational therapy evaluation also supported the results of the psychological and speech and language evaluation. Bob was somewhat underresponsive to sound, including speech. He liked visual detail and had difficulty completing tasks when there was a lot of visual stimulation present. The confusion that Bob experienced when presented with a great deal of visual stimulation led to contact gestures to protest and then eventually to tantrum behavior including aggression and self-injurious behavior.

The results of the Functional Analysis appeared to bring all parts of the evaluation together to help explain Bob's aggression and self-injury. In terms of environmental conditions, his behaviors occurred at a very high rate during tabletop activities, particularly when there were a number of objects on the table. The behavior problems very rarely occurred during leisure when Bob could play with his cars or out on the playground. Bob's behavior problems seem to occur more frequently when he had not slept well at night. They also occurred more frequently during allergy season in which pollen levels were high. In terms of the functions of Bob's aggressive behaviors, parents reported that they felt the behaviors were often used to escape difficult tasks. Parents noted that Bob would frequently begin to look away from a task. He would then use a contact gesture to take the person's hand, and move the tasks away. If this were unsuccessful, Bob would become very frustrated and display aggression or self-injury.

The results of the evaluation led to a number of recommendations for Bob that would enhance his ability to learn functional skills, as well as help him manage his aggressive behaviors. One of the primary recommendations was to put a visual schedule in effect. The purpose of the visual schedule was to show Bob activities that were upcoming, and to convey expectancies to him. This was put in place partially because of Bob's difficulty understanding language. A visual schedule was also arranged so that less desirable activities during the day were always followed by highly desirable activities. This visually portrayed to Bob that if he could get through some of the tabletop activities that he could engage in free play with his cars or go outside.

Another recommendation revolved around how to arrange the tabletop activities so that they would reduce protest behaviors. For example, it was recommended that only one item was to be placed on the table. When there was a series of tasks to complete, they would be placed in a "work box," and when they were completed they went into a "finished box." This was done so that Bob could see his progress toward earning his reward of a reinforcing activity. In addition to the above recommendations, the speech and language pathologist recommended that Bob learn a communicative response that would represent asking for help on tasks that were too difficult for him. He also was to be taught a protest response that would appropriately request a brief break from activities when they became overwhelming, or when his attention span wasn't sufficient to attend any longer.

In addition to the above recommendations, emerging skills were selected from the psycho-educational profile and the Vineland. These skills were seen as very important by Bob's parents and those working with him at school. Since they were skills that Bob had almost mastered, he was motivated to learn them and there was less protesting because of putting him in situations that were too difficult for him.

Editors' Note:

Vellet and Reese provide an excellent overview of issues facing today's psychologist working in team settings. Of particular interest was the discussion of potential func-

tional purposes served by aberrant behavior. In the last twenty years, professionals have gradually begun to view behavior in something other than a negative light. The editors support the position forwarded by Vellet and Reese that we all need to be acutely in tune with the potential communicative and other purposes served by children's behavior.

REFERENCES

Achenbach, T. M. (1991). *Child behavior checklist 4-18.* Burlington, VT: University of Vermont Department of Psychiatry.

Achenbach, T. M. (1991). *Youth self-report 11-18.* Burlington, VT: University of Vermont Department of Psychiatry.

American Psychiatric Association. (1994). *Diagnostic and statistical manual of mental disorders* (4th ed.). Washington, D.C.: Author.

Bailey, J. M., Pyles, O. A. M. (1989). Behavioral diagnostics. In E. Cipiani (ed.) *The treatment of severe behavior disorders.* (pp. 85-107). Washington, D.C.: American Association on Mental Retardation.

Bayley, N. (1993). *Bayley scales of infant development* (2nd. ed.). San Antonio, TX. The Psychological Corporation, Harcourt, Brace, & Company.

Bene, E. (1985). *Family relations test.* London: The National Foundation for Educational Research in England and Wales.

Carlson, C. I. (1990). Assessing the family context. In C. R. Reynolds and R. W. Kamphaus (Eds.) *Handbook of psychological and educational assessment of children: Personality, behavior, and context.* New York: The Guilford Press.

Dunst, C. J., Trivette, C. M., & Deal, A. G. (Eds.). (1994). Supporting & strengthening families: Volume 1: *Methods, strategies, and practices.* Cambridge, MA: Brookline.

Durand, V. M., & Crimmins, D. B. (1988). Identifying the variables maintaining self-injurious behavior. *Journal of Autism and Developmental Disorders, 18,* 99-117.

Erikson, J. (1997). The infant-toddler developmental assessment (IDA): A family-centered transdisciplinary assessment process. In S. M. Meisels & E. Fenichel (Eds.) *New visions for the developmental assessment of infants and young children.* Washington, DC: Zero to Three: National Center for Infants, Toddlers, and Families.

Grossman, H. J. (Ed.). (1983). *Classification in mental retardation.* Washington, DC: American Association on Mental Deficiency.

Harter, S. (1985). *Self-perception profile for children.* Denver, CO: University of Denver Press.

Jastak, S. (1993). *Wide range achievement test-third edition.* Wilmington, DE: Jastak Associates, Inc.

Kaufman, A. S., & Kaufman, N. L. (1983). *Kaufman assessment battery for children.* Circle Pines, MN: American Guidance Service.

Kaufman, A. S., & Kaufman, N. L. (1985). *Kaufman test of educational achievement.* Circle Pines, MN: American Guidance Service.

Kovacs, M. (1982). *Children's depression inventory.* Toronto: Multi-Health Systems, Inc.

Leiter, R. G. (1948). *Leiter international performance scale.* Chicago: Stoelting Co.

Lincoln, A. J., Kaufman, J., & Kaufman, A. S. (1995). Intellectual and cognitive assessment. In M. Hersen & R. T. Ammerman (Eds.), *Advanced abnormal child psychology.* Hillsdale, NJ, Lawrence Erlbaum.

McArthur, D. S., & Roberts, G. E. (1982). *Roberts apperception test for children.* Los Angeles: Western Psychological Services.

Meisels, S. J., & Fenichel, E. (1997). *New visions for the developmental assessment of infants and young children.* Washington, DC: Zero to Three: National Center for Infants, Toddlers, and Families.

Moos, R. H., & Moos, B. S. (1986). *Family environment scale* (2nd ed.). Palo Alto, CA: Consulting Psychologists Press, Inc.

Olson, D. H., Portner, J., & Lavee, Y. (1985). *Family adaptability & cohesion evaluation scales.* St. Paul, MN: Family Social Science, University of Minnesota.

O'Neill, R. E., Horner, R. H., Albin, R. W., Storey, K., & Sprague, J. R. (1990). *Functional analysis of problem behavior: A practical assessment guide.* Pacific Grove, CA: Brooks/Cole.

Reichard, A. (1997). Parent and professional perspectives on elements of an effective visit to a program that provides educational and clinical services to children with developmental and related disabilities. Unpublished manuscript.

Reynolds, C. R., & Richmond, B. O. (1985). *Revised Children's Manifest Anxiety Scale.* Los Angeles, CA.: Western Psychological Services.

Sattler, J. M. (1992). *Assessment of Children* (3rd ed.). San Diego: author.

Schopler, E., & Reichler, R. J. (1979). Individualized assessment and treatment for autistic and developmentally disabled children: Volume I: *Psychoeducational profile.* Baltimore: University Park Press.

Sparrow, S. S., Balla, D. A., & Cicchetti, D. V. (1984). *Vineland adaptive behavior scales, Interview edition, survey form.* Circle Pines, Minnesota: American Guidance Service.

Wechsler, D. (1989). *Wechsler preschool and primary scale of intelligence-Revised.* San Antonio, TX. The Psychological Corporation; Harcourt, Brace, & Jovanovich, Inc.

Wechsler, D. (1991). *Wechsler intelligence scale for children-Third edition.* San Antonio, TX. The Psychological Corporation; Harcourt, Brace, & Jovanovich, Inc.

Woodcock, R. W. (1977). *Woodcock-Johnson psychoeducational battery.* Allen, TX: DLM Teaching Resources.

Chapter 14

SCHOOL COUNSELING

FRANCES PALMER, MARY DECK AND DALE BROTHERTON

MAJOR ROLES AND RESPONSIBILITIES OF
SCHOOL COUNSELORS

Many parents who have had little or no contact with their child's school counseling program automatically assume one of two things about today's school counselor. First, they may associate the school counselor with their high school counselor of one or two decades past and their memories of this person as one who scheduled classes, provided information about college and possibly careers, and kept records of credits for graduation. Or, they may envision the school counselor as someone similar to the stereotype of a psychiatrist, who is privy to the deepest, darkest secrets of children and adolescents and who, consequently, is in somewhat of an adversarial relationship with parents. Both of these misconceptions tend to deter parents from utilizing the school counselor's trained helping skills and unique position within the educational setting to their advantage. However, once the contact is made and a helping relationship is established between the parents and the school counselor, the result is usually one that benefits all parties, primarily the child or adolescent involved.

School counseling is a relatively young profession that emerged from the vocational guidance movement of the early 1900s (Schmidt, 1996). Unlike other counselors who serve a target audience, such as marriage counselors or drug and alcohol abuse counselors, the school counselor provides multiple services most often to three populations: students, parents, and teachers. Certification through each state's department of education is a condition for practicing school counselors, with periodic renewal of credentials required. In most states, the minimum educational level is a master's degree program, in which the counselor-in-training participates in graduate courses in such areas as human development, special education, psychology, career assessment and development, test and measurement techniques, ethics, educational research, and counseling processes and theories (Schmidt, 1996). This broad base of training includes many of the same courses required for establishing a private practice in counseling and prepares the counselor for the variety of services offered to students, parents, and teachers. One study (Paisley & Hubbard, 1989) indicates that twenty-nine states also specify teaching experience before certification and/or employment as a school counselor. The experience and education required of school counselors uniquely qualify them to "bridge the gap" between the school system and the family system.

The term "school counseling" describes both the profession and the program of services established by counselors in schools. As used in this chapter, "counseling" refers to a wide selection of services and activities that counselors choose to help people prevent disabling events, focus on their overall development, and remedy existing concerns. The purpose of a school counseling program is to provide a variety of services that facilitate the total development—educational, career, personal, and social—of all students through a comprehensive program developed in response to identified needs, goals, and objectives of the school and community (Schmidt, 1996).

Above all else, the school counselor serves as the "student advocate," a role which assumes promoting the best interests of the student at all times. The school counselor may be the only person in the school who knows each child on the school campus by name and knows his or her particular needs and background. This personal relationship makes the school counselor a partner with the parent rather than an adversary.

The first contact parents have with the school counselor may result from educational concerns they have about their child. American schools have made giant strides in providing an equal, appropriate, and effective education for all children. The school counselor's role in the educational development of the child includes assessment of students' abilities and specific needs, placement of students in appropriate instructional programs based on this assessment and other data, coordination of opportunities for parents to monitor their child's academic progress, and the counseling of students about their academic and career goals (Schmidt, 1996). School counselors welcome and encourage parental involvement in planning the child's academic instructional program. A discussion of the role of the school counselor and parents in conjunction with other instructional personnel in the coordination and development of the child's instructional program will follow in the later sections of this chapter.

Although facilitating the student's educational potential is a primary function of the school counselor, most counselors realize that students, just like adults, have needs and/or problems which affect their performance. Studies in child and adolescent growth and development indicate predictable stages of potential growth and crises. The school counselor, through a comprehensive classroom guidance program endorsed by the school and community, initiates strategies to address problems which may appear at specific stages of development, such as handling peer pressure and learning the effects of tobacco, drug, and alcohol abuse (middle school and high school), adjusting to new school settings (first year of middle school and high school and transfer students), learning how to make friends (elementary grades), acquiring skills of conflict resolution (all grades), making good choices (all grades), and learning to respect others who are different (all grades). These skills may be taught by the counselor in the classroom setting or by the classroom teacher with direction by the counselor.

In addition to stage/age conflicts, individual students will inevitably face personal and emotional issues which can adversely affect academic progress. Brain research now tells us that "emotion is a very important educative process because it drives attention, which drives learning and memory" (Sylwester, 1995, p. 72). Serious problems might include how to deal with the effects of sexual and physical abuse, parental divorce or abandonment, or the death of a significant person or even a pet, all of which may lead to thoughts of suicide for some students. Certainly, the school counselor is duty-bound by law to report suspected cases of abuse or neglect to appropriate agencies and to notify parents or guardians about specific suicidal ideation or injury to self or others. Once the legal aspects have been addressed, the counselor may refer the child (and parents) to outside sources.

In addition to these serious emotional concerns, studies have shown that group and individual counseling within the school setting can be very effective in teaching students how to cope with these issues and others of a less traumatic nature, such as test anxiety, organization skills, and goal setting (Borders & Drury, 1992; Myrick & Dixon, 1985; Omizo & Omizo, 1987). Most counselors require students interested in participating in group counseling with other students experiencing similar problems to have a parent or guardian give permission for participation.

Many school counselors also provide opportunities for parent training programs or parent advocacy groups for interested parents. These programs are usually developed in response to parental requests and are generally offered outside the school day to accommodate the schedules of working parents. Many outstanding programs have been in existence for some time so that the counselor can serve as the facilitator of an already successful program. Furthermore, school counselors reach out to parents through newsletters, telephone conferences, or by arranging meetings with teachers and administrators upon the parents' request.

Although school counselors, especially at the high school level, still do work with scheduling, college entrance, and credits for graduation, the role of the school counselor has dramatically changed over the past few decades. Perhaps this brief introduction is a beginning in clarifying the role of today's school counselor to parents and other adults interested in the school counseling program. However, there cannot be an effective school counseling program without a collaborative effort among the school counselor, the parents, and other professionals within the school and community. The school counselor, albeit well-trained and sensitive to students, cannot, without help from others, adequately serve the diverse needs of all students in the school setting where the ratio is most often one counselor to every five hundred students. Thus, an interdisciplinary approach is optimal in meeting these needs.

CONTRIBUTIONS OF SCHOOL COUNSELING TO INTERDISCIPLINARY PRACTICE

Participation in interdisciplinary teams is not new to school counselors, and such involvement is likely to grow (Greer, Greer, & Woody, 1995). Since the passage of the Education for All Handicapped Children Act of 1975, counselors have joined with parents, special education teachers, educational diagnosticians, regular education teachers, school administrators, and other helping professionals (possibly including but not limited to speech pathologists, assistive technologists, physical therapists, occupational therapists, physicians, psychologists, and social workers) in the development of the Individualized Education Programs (IEPs) for special education students. With the more recent Education for Handicapped Amendments (Public Law 99-457) in 1986, the counselor also participates in the team's development of the Individualized Family Service Plan (IFSP). In both instances, the team can be most often coordinated by, if not officially headed by, the school counselor due to their familiarity with the child and his or her special needs (Greer et al., 1995).

Because the school counselor is best acquainted with the many factors in a child's family and school system, the counselor can often make sense of all of the "loose ends" reported by other professionals. In most cases, prior to referral for assessment, the counselor and the classroom teacher(s) have already discussed and attempted modifications. Finding that these attempts are not successful, the counselor is usually the one to follow the referral process from beginning to end, by helping the parent or regular education teacher initiate the paperwork; collecting data from school records, parents, teachers, and other professionals; observing student behavior and performance; notifying classroom teachers of assessment times; and providing input during the IEP committee (student placement committee) meeting, a process which is repeated at least once every three years.

One result of the referral process is the close communication which develops between the parents and the school counselor. Often when the IEP committee convenes, the parents may experience unintentional intimidation, even though they may be acquainted with each professional involved. The counselor possesses the skill to foster and maintain an atmosphere of trust and open communication among all members of the team and to make the parents feel that they are an integral part of the decision-making process (Greer et al., 1995). Since the counselor's role is that of student advocate, he or she becomes the liaison between the parents and school personnel. The counselor's specific training in communication skills can help provide an emotional environment that would be as nonthreatening as possible to all participants.

As inclusion becomes more widely practiced within school districts so that children with disabilities are served within the regular education classroom, the school counselor will need to become more knowledgeable of children with severe disabilities. Counselors can turn to the interdisciplinary experts, such as physicians, occupational therapists, and physical therapists, as well as parents, to familiarize themselves with the unique problems facing the student with special needs. Often the student cannot or is unwilling to express needs which result from his or her disability, especially one that is physical in nature. Therefore, the counselor must depend on the experts from the interdisciplinary team to provide insights. For example, an occupational therapist in one district arranged several times during the summer for a student with an orthopedic disability to have a tour of the school building and visit with the school counselor and some of the teachers before the student entered sixth grade. The self-confidence this new sixth grader gained through these tours was immeasurable and resulted in much less stress in the fall when school began. Similarly, classroom teachers need to be prepared for students with disabilities who are assigned to their classes. Since the school counselor generally works with the scheduling needs of students with disabilities to be certain that their IEP is followed, the counselor could be the one to meet with these teachers in an in-service training program prior to the opening of classes. The obvious benefit would be a smoother beginning to the year for the student and the teacher.

Unfortunately, few teacher education programs provide in-depth training in special education for regular education teachers. Although this trend is changing, veteran teachers have had little or no special education instruction, which inevitably leads to frustration among everyone. For this reason, the counselor, along with special education teachers and other professionals from the interdisciplinary team, can arrange and provide in-service programs tailored to fit the needs of the specific campus and its special education population. In addition, when the professionals provide up-to-date information regarding effective classroom strategies, the counselor can disseminate this information to school personnel directly involved with a particular student. This direct contact between, for instance, physicians and teachers with the school counselor as liaison provides factual information in an efficient manner. For example, when a student with Tourette Syndrome entered one school last year, few teachers were familiar with this disorder, and problems were certain to occur due to ignorance. Although the physician could not actually come to the school, he provided the school counselor with current information regarding Tourette's Syndrome and suggested classroom modifications in dealing with this student, which the school counselor, in turn, relayed to the student's teachers. After reading the material, the instructional team met with the parent, special education teacher, and the school counselor to decide how to provide this student with the most appropriate educational opportunities. The results, using collaboration, were much more successful than a trial-and-error approach in serving this child.

The school counselor and educators of exceptional children tend to form a close collaborative relationship as they deal with the needs of special students on a daily basis. Counselors depend on these special education teachers to provide the most recent interpretations of federal laws which affect the special education programs and to make counselors aware of any special needs the exceptional child may have. The counselor could meet with special education teachers daily for the first three weeks of school to determine the success of the students' placements and to anticipate any problems which may require a new IEP committee meeting. For example, on one campus the special education teachers provide modifications for all teachers and meet with the grade level teams and administrators to discuss the special circumstances of each student on their caseload. Then, the counselor can assist the special education teacher with support and understanding needed to work with these students on a daily basis. For example, some students with behavior modification plans are allowed to leave the special education setting to work on the school counselor's office computer or to run errands as part of their reward system. Working together always increases appreciation for the job performed by other professionals.

Another important role of the interdisciplinary team is to offer support and help to parents and guardians of children with special needs. Parents of exceptional children face obstacles unknown to most parents. This is particularly true of students who have a debilitating mental, emotional, or physical disability. The guilt sometimes associated with having a child with any type of disability, combined with the challenges of daily care, supervision, and parenting, often seems insurmountable (Schmidt, 1996). The interdisciplinary team can be available to answer questions and hear suggestions from these parents. Because of the federal funds and the legal issues involved in serving special education students, the team also has the responsibility of making parents aware of their rights and the rights of their child and ensuring that these rights are protected in the educational setting. Finally, the counselor, along with other team members, can provide referral information regarding parent support groups and helping agencies within the community, as well as coordinating such groups for parents of exceptional students within the school itself.

THE ROLES PARENTS TYPICALLY PLAY IN OPTIMAL INTERDISCIPLINARY SERVICE PROVISION OF SCHOOL COUNSELING

Without a doubt, the most important role of the parents is to stay in close communication with the interdisciplinary team, often through the school counselor, regarding their child's education. Through the referral and/or placement process, parents and the school counselor have already established a relationship of trust and mutual respect. Since the counselor may function as the liaison between parents and the interdisciplinary team, most parental contact will initiate with the counselor. It is extremely important that the parents of special education students develop a rapport with the school counselor before any problems occur. This enables an opening of communication paths and opportunities to establish a trusting parent/counselor relationship. In general, most parents of exceptional students are the first to become aware of problems at school, as evidenced by the following example. Within a week after the opening of school, the school counselor received a call from a parent of an eighth grader who has a pervasive developmental disorder and exhibits limited speech ability. Although Dusty (not his real name) appeared to know the school counselor well and always greeted her with a big hug, he could not tell her that he was unhappy, but his mother knew. He began to exhibit somatic complaints of nausea and dreaded coming to school, a reaction which was entirely out of character. It was Dusty's mother who determined that he was unhappy because his new schedule did not permit him to eat lunch with his best friend, a girl in the Life Skills class. The team immediately called a placement committee meeting with his teachers and administrators to determine a change in scheduling so that Dusty could be with his friend at lunch. This simple change restored the boy's love of school and further cemented the bond between this sensitive, insightful mother and the interdisciplinary team.

Not all problems are this easy to remedy, however, so parents must be familiar with the federal laws that relate to their rights as stated in the Individual with Disabilities Education Act (IDEA) or Section 504 of the

Rehabilitation Act of 1973. Parental rights and responsibilities must be presented in a written format to all parents of children referred for special education assessment, and most parents find that they have many copies of this document since they receive a copy at each yearly IEP meeting. However, many parents do not "do their homework" regarding federal laws and simply trust the school to abide by federal guidelines. Unless the parents are familiar with these guidelines and are equally familiar with their child's IEP, it is possible for even well-intentioned school personnel to be remiss in their duties. When a parent recognizes that certain IEP modifications for the child are not being implemented, it is the parent's responsibility to report this inequity to a member of the interdisciplinary team (most likely the school counselor). The school counselor often may be the ideal liaison between the parent and the regular education teacher. Many times, though, the parent feels most comfortable talking directly with the counselor or special education teacher first.

Most of these contacts will occur soon after the opening of school when parents have had a chance to receive input from their child. For instance, a parent of a student with learning disabilities called one school counselor with a concern that her son's pre-algebra teacher was not following the modifications in the child's IEP. Because the school counselor knew that the student's special education teacher had already distributed copies of the IEP to the regular education teachers, she called a conference with the math teacher and the special education teacher. They discussed classroom modifications for this student who had really blossomed since his learning disability had been identified in the preceding year. The math teacher, who was new to the district, admitted that he had not read all of the modifications on the special education students in his classes. The school counselor and the special education teacher pointed out to him as stated in the IEP that in addition to his specific learning disability in math, this boy has developmental dyslexia (or) also a learning disability in reading, a condition which had been affecting his performance in pre-algebra. It was as if a light had come on for the teacher, and he learned a valuable lesson about becoming familiar with his students' IEPs. Had the parent not been aware of the problem, however, this child could have gone for weeks without appropriate interventions. He might have failed for the term, thus causing him to be ineligible for football, a potentially devastating blow to his self-esteem. This familiarity with the child's IEP is even more crucial for parents of elementary students or students with more severe disabilities who cannot express problems occurring within the regular classroom to their parents. In short, parents must be the watchdog of their child's rights and must assert these rights until they are provided.

A year earlier, the parent to whom the same school counselor referred in the preceding vignette would have stormed up to the school and tearfully demanded to see the school counselor, the principal, the superintendent, and the special education director about the "abuse" to her child. What she has learned and what all parents, especially those parents of exceptional children, might remember is an old adage, "you kill more flies with honey than with vinegar."

School counselors have received training and are equipped to model openness, respect, and acceptance of others' points of view, all of which foster a collaborative spirit between parents and members of the interdisciplinary team. Parents who practice these same techniques will ensure the best results for their child. Taking time to facilitate an understanding of what it is like to have an exceptional child enables parents to provide insight and foster empathy for their position and requests. Similarly, educators can help parents understand what it is like to be responsible for 150 students every day and sincerely seek to meet the needs of each child, knowing the virtual impossibility of such a task. Meeting with the interdisciplinary team to discuss such issues before a crisis arises can pave the way for greater cooperation when and if one does happen. All parents of special education and students identified under Section 504 of the Rehabilitation Act of 1975 are encouraged to have a team conference within two weeks after the opening of school to prepare the teachers for the special needs of their child. Most teachers welcome any background information which can prove insightful when dealing with the exceptional children in their care. When the parent does not initiate such action, it can be recommended by the interdisciplinary team and arranged by the school counselor.

An additional important role of the interdisciplinary team could be to provide suggestions for the families of the exceptional child. Although often underutilized, members of the team possess a wealth of knowledge and experience which could benefit the family system. Recommendations might include treatment options, including pharmacological therapy, from the physician on the team, and input regarding successful behavior modification or intervention techniques as suggested by the team psychologist. Certainly, the professional educators could suggest strategies for optimal success in completing homework, studying for tests, and learning organization skills. Of course, the school counselor might add coping strategies for family members in dealing with the exceptional child. School counselors have had experience in discussing somewhat sensitive issues such as sexual awareness on a one-on-one basis with students. Often parents are unprepared or unwilling to educate their child about issues such as menstruation, for example. The parent may feel comfortable in relegating this role to the counselor, especially if it is affecting the child's performance in school in some way. Another option would be for the parent and the counselor to talk with the child together when addressing such sensitive areas. This intervention can also build trust with the child or adolescent to feel comfortable in approaching the school counselor, should other concerns of a sensitive nature arise. Such interventions should convince the family that they are not alone in their struggles and that there is a source of concerned support available to them when needed.

Finally, parents can improve the productivity of the interdisciplinary team by keeping abreast of current information regarding their child's disability or medical condition. This knowledge can provide understanding and insights as well as an awareness of up-to-date research findings, treatment options, and modifications for their child's condition. School counselors appreciate parents who share such information, which they then can relate to the other team members who will be directly involved in the child's education. In addition, parents of exceptional children can further increase their awareness by becoming involved in local and state associations and by attending conferences of these organizations. Although economic considerations may forego some of the prior suggestions, parents can always visit the public library, talk with team professionals, or attend free parent support group meetings. Being armed with knowledge can only serve to improve the effectiveness of the interdisciplinary approach as well as the parents' desire to ensure their child's best interests.

TYPICAL PARENT QUESTIONS/COMMENTS FOR
SCHOOL COUNSELING

I am frustrated when professionals don't listen to parents. A teacher or other professional may have more experience with children in general, but parents spend much more time interacting with their specific child. What advice would you give your peers to encourage them to listen to parents? How can I tactfully confront a professional if I don't think they are listening?

Your feelings of frustration are certainly understandable. It sounds as though you have had one or more unpleasant experiences with your child's teacher or some other professional involved in his or her education. Other parents have also expressed this concern (see Chapter 2). You specifically request advice for other school professionals which would encourage them to listen to parents. If you are referring to an experience with a regular education teacher, one reason for this apparent inability to listen to parents may be, as explained earlier, that many regular education teachers have had little or no formal training in special education. If this is the case, arrange for an informal meeting with the teacher(s) and include the counselor and special education teacher. Prior to this meeting, discuss your concerns with the special education personnel involved with your child and with the school counselor in order to determine a strategy to best approach the teachers. The school counselor has training in mediation techniques and is in the unique position to understand the total situation. The counselor and special education teacher are probably personally acquainted with your child as well and can share insights gained in working with him or her.

To prevent this situation from occurring in the future, establish a positive rapport with school personnel in advance of a crisis situation, as suggested earlier in the chapter. Once again, your school counselor is trained in techniques to foster mutual respect and understanding. When school personnel know of your concerns and prior problems within the setting of a non-threatening team conference, they are more likely to be open to listen to your suggestions and to be more understanding if problems do arise.

The answer to the second question is dependent upon the mutual trust, respect, and openness previously established. A negative approach can destroy the best intentions and alienate you and your child from those who could be of great help. As the parent of the exceptional child, you are your child's strongest advocate. Remember that most of the school personnel are also parents themselves, and the appeal from this perspective best provides realization about your unique situation. Use the "honey" approach with a prearranged strategy determined by you, the school counselor, and any other trusted member of the interdisciplinary team. The team approach in this situation is usually quite effective because of the variety of input afforded by the professionals in the group. Maintain a concerned, yet assertive attitude, with your focus always on the welfare of your child.

Counselors experienced in working with parents of exceptional children have found that a positive, cooperative approach is most effective. They attend the annual IEP committee meetings of all of the students who are or who will be attending their campuses. Attending students' IEP meetings provides school counselors the opportunity to work with the parents and the entire team regarding the child's best interests. As a parent, establish an optimal collaborative relationship with all of the personnel who will directly interact with your child in the school year.

If for some reason you do not feel that a teacher or other educator is listening to your concerns, especially after you have tried an informal conference, you may wish to convene an IEP committee to discuss your concerns. Although this may be construed by some as somewhat threatening, the IEP meeting provides a structured forum for your child's interests. Again, your approach should be collaborative rather than adversarial, but you can be certain that the educational personnel will be attuned to your concerns in this format.

Dr. Schulz' Response:

Open communication cannot be stressed enough. One parent revealed her feelings on attending her first IEP meeting. She said, "The teacher, the principal, and the psychologist were all seated on one side of the table and my chair was placed facing them. I knew I didn't have a chance of getting my point across." Unless the parent is perceived as a team member there is no valid communication and certainly no positive result.

My son's disability isn't the problem. Dealing with the denial of family members and school personnel has been the problem. Do you have advice specific to dealing with denial?

Although you do not indicate your son's specific disability, by your statement, his disability sounds like one that may have few or no obvious outward physical manifestations. It could be a specific learning disability or a behavioral disorder, such as Attention Deficit Disorder (with or without Hyperactivity), both of which appear in otherwise "normal" children, who may, in fact, have above-average intelligence. Although behavioral disorders almost always become evident in the elementary grades, often a child is able to mask a learning disability until the curriculum becomes more difficult in middle school. Because of these facts, some adults tend to discount these problems as ones that could be fixed if the child would simply try harder. Unfortunately, educational professionals and the general public, including family members, who would never hesitate to provide compassion and assistance to those who are orthopedically impaired, for example, are sometimes less accommodating to children with disabilities which are not obvious in appearance.

However, these hidden disabilities are just as debilitating and frustrating as the more obvious physical ones. Education is the key to acceptance and eventual understanding of these conditions. In many school districts, counselors and special education personnel provide literature which helps explain the inherent problems in such disabilities. Ideally, attendance at a conference which focuses in the areas of concern could be recommended to family members. Hearing from experts tends to give more credibility to what you have been saying all along. If this is not feasible, family members could attend family support groups or visit with the school counselor about the problem. Suggest to your school counselor the possibility of developing parent/family training programs. Your school counselor can be an invaluable resource in this area.

When you sense denial of school personnel regarding your son's disability, contact your school counselor (assuming he or she is not the one in denial) and special education personnel as well as others on the interdisciplinary team to assist you in disseminating information regarding your child's problem. The counselor has probably worked closely with the school personnel in question at other times and has developed rapport so that suggestions may be more accepted coming from the counselor. Oftentimes, federal monies are available for school personnel to attend special education conferences about the different kinds of disabilities. Be on the lookout for such conferences, and feel free to recommend them to the educational personnel at your school. Remember that only the most recent graduates of teacher education programs have significant training in special education issues, and any literature you can provide for your child's teachers is usually appreciated and studied. Talk with your school administrators about requiring training in the needs of all special children in your school system and be available for suggestions from a parent's perspective regarding this training. Once again, it cannot be stressed enough that you request a team conference with the more stubborn members of your child's instructional team after a strategy session with your school counselor, special education teacher, and more open-minded members of the team.

Finally, you may wish to initiate a counseling relationship with a family counselor. In fact, your school counselor could provide referrals for such counselors in your area. Perspective from an outside, concerned source may be exactly what you and your family need. This counselor could work with the family dynamics, including denial, relating to your child with a disability. Furthermore, a family counselor can help you to discover strategies to become a more effective advocate for your child as you deal with the school system.

Dr. Schulz's Response:

When parents who have children with disabilities are overwhelmed with their tasks and responsibilities, meeting with other parents can be especially helpful. Sometimes it just helps to know that "the grass is browner on the other side" and sometimes parents can share strategies they have found to be helpful.

My child's condition has truly affected our family. Comparing her with "regular" kids her age in daycare, with friends, at local playgrounds has been difficult. In addition, the need to research and network with others and realizing you cannot trust doctors to do the right thing generates ongoing stress. I now feel I must maintain a career with flexibility and consider only those family moves that can accommodate my daughter's medical and other needs. I'm also not enthusiastic about family travel and other activities of typical

family life. Furthermore, I feel like I don't have enough time for my children or my spouse. The most difficult thing is wondering what my daughter will be like, how far she will go. I worry about her future and her family's future.

You have very eloquently expressed the concerns of all parents who have children with severe disabilities. Your frustration and worry clearly have overwhelmed you, which has obviously affected the normal life most families take for granted. Unfortunately, you have also had an unsatisfactory experience with your daughter's doctors, which has left you with no professional whom you can trust and to whom you can express your concerns, both medical and emotional. However, although your frustration is obvious, so is your unmistakable love for your child and your family. Between the lines, there appear two things: your desire to make everything all right for your daughter and your family and also your perceived incompetence at balancing all your roles of parent, provider, and spouse.

You're right. Your life has radically changed, and it will never be the same as it once was because of your child's disability. Every decision you make from now on must be weighed against her needs. But remember that your life also radically changed when you married and when you had your other children. It is apparent that you consider their needs as well, in every decision you make. Stop being so hard on yourself. You may not be aware of this, but every caring parent feels the same way you do, even ones who do not have children with disabilities. Your child's disability is not your fault, nor is it hers. Do what you can and all that you can, but realize that you cannot do it all. You are only human; be realistic about your limitations and accept them. What advice would you give to a parent in the same situation? Think about it, and then take your own advice.

As much as is expedient, strive to give each member of your family, including yourself, a life that is as nearly normal as possible, but don't try to shoulder this immense responsibility by yourself; it must be a family affair. What is it that you would love to do if you had spare time? Make time for that activity. Since so many obviously depend on you, don't neglect yourself, as the super-parent tendency suggests. Take care of your own health issues just as you do for your children. Being rested and healthy gives you more energy to deal with your every day stresses more efficiently.

One of the greatest areas of stress in families where there is a child with a disability is between the husband and wife. Nurture this relationship just as you are obviously doing with your child with a disability. For example, plan a date every month and a weekend getaway twice a year. Granted, this takes a great deal of planning to find a trusted sitter and to make other arrangements. But, it will pay off in a closer, more committed relationship with your spouse through the difficult times you are certain to encounter, and it will provide you both an opportunity to set family priorities. It also provides a wonderful example for your children.

Your children without disabilities also need your time. Often, these children are unintentionally neglected in favor of the sibling with a disability. Prioritize your time so that you or your spouse spends time alone each week with each child. This should be fun time, in addition to the time you spend doing homework, watching TV, and going to church or community events. It is imperative that each child respect and value the differences of your daughter, and the best way to teach this is through modeling. Going on family outings is not easy, but it is so important for your family so that they and others see your desire to provide a normal life for all of your children. Bring along a sitter or another family member to do the little extras which may otherwise prevent you from enjoying these times together as a family.

You state that you know you need to network, and I would encourage you to set aside time to share with other parents who have successfully walked the path you have begun. These parents are more than willing to assist you with emotional support and coping strategies. It sounds as if you are in a metropolitan area. If so, your local phone directory will list parent support groups. Depending on your child's disability, you may want to contact your doctor, hospital, school district, or mental health agency to locate a parent network. The internet is loaded with sources, too. You mention the need to do research. A parent support group that is already well established will be able to provide you with literature and current research, thus freeing you from this job. Although locating and participating in a parent support group may sound like one more unnecessary responsibility, believe me, it will be worth it in the long run.

You do not state the actual disability, so it is next to impossible to estimate her specific educational and social prognosis. However, your daughter will probably progress farther than you now believe is possible, simply because of the advances and opportunities that will emerge in the next few decades for children with disabilities. You can explore every avenue for success for her and even become an advocate for children with disabilities in the school and community. Yes, you will make mistakes in child rearing, but everyone does. Redirect your natural worry into action for your child and your family. There are parents who have children with disabilities who lead the most fulfilled lives of all parents, and your concern indicates that this will be the case for you as well.

Dr. Schulz's Response:

This issue may be the most difficult one we face as parents of children with disabilities. I once read about a mother who said, in referring to her son who had men-

tal retardation, "I gave him my life." Her daughters replied, "And we gave him our mother." We tend to be martyrs, an unattractive and boring role. Over the years I have developed the ability to say, "I'm doing the best I can. I need a break!" And I'm talking to myself.

CASE EXAMPLE

The following case example illustrates specific times and interventions across the elementary school years when the school counselor provided direct services through a developmental school counseling program to a child with mild mental disabilities. The services included parent and teacher consultation, classroom guidance, individual and small group counseling, and peer helper training.

Before Chris entered kindergarten, his parents had observed that he was slower at learning some things than his older siblings had been. They had taken Chris to a child development clinic where Chris was evaluated as having a mild mental disability that would require some special attention when Chris began school, particularly in the areas of fine motor skills, ability to focus on tasks, and academic skills. When Chris's parents registered Chris for kindergarten, they were introduced to teachers and staff, including the school counselor. The school counselor distributed a pamphlet to parents explaining the responsibilities of the elementary school counselor and invited them to use these services. Chris's parents took the time to introduce themselves to the school counselor and to inquire briefly whether the school counselor would also be working with children like Chris. The school counselor assured them of being available for them and for Chris and that the counselor would be working with all the children in the school.

When Chris began kindergarten, the school counselor attended the IEP (Individual Education Program) meeting with Chris's parents and others members of the school team to specify how Chris's school needs would be met. The parents learned that the school counselor would be going into all kindergarten classrooms periodically for classroom guidance and focusing on learning skills (listening and following directions), social skills (sharing and making friends), and expressive skills (identifying and naming feelings). It was determined that at this time Chris would require no additional interventions by the counselor. When the school counselor went into the kindergarten classes to lead the classroom guidance lessons, the counselor's awareness of Chris's needs allowed the counselor to plan several specific strategies to ensure that Chris was included in the activities and was successful.

During the first grade, Chris was placed in a resource room each day for reading and math and remained in the general classroom the remainder of the day. Chris's primary contact with the school counselor continued to be through regularly scheduled classroom guidance sessions. However, in the second grade, when Chris exhibited increased frustration with the schedule and expectations in the regular second grade, the counselor assumed a more active role in working with Chris. Chris seemed anxious in the mornings before coming to school, cried at times when asked to complete tasks by the regular class teacher, and was often resistant to returning to the regular classroom from the resource room. The school counselor consulted with the regular and special education teachers and Chris's parents about Chris's problems. Through consultation, they agreed that changes in Chris's classroom routines and the provision of a volunteer tutor to help Chris two days a week in the regular class would be useful. It was also decided that the counselor would include Chris in a small counseling group designed to help first and second graders with stress management. The counselor also provided the parents with information on stress management techniques for them to try at home with Chris. Chris's frustration and stress were significantly reduced through these interventions.

When Chris was in the third grade, the family experienced a house fire during a holiday break from school. The fire occurred at night when no one was home except Chris and his mother. They were not harmed, but the fire so damaged the house that the family had to move out temporarily and move in with the relatives. On the first day back from the break, the school counselor met with Chris's mother who told her that Chris had been having trouble sleeping, talked constantly about the fire, and was fearful when out of the mother's sight for any length of time. To help reduce Chris's fears and anxieties related to the fire, they decided that the counselor would see Chris for individual counseling for four weeks, twice a week for 30 minutes each session. Using play therapy, story telling, and bibliotherapy, and by reviewing with Chris stress management techniques previously learned, the counselor helped Chris reduce his fears and worries about the fire. Chris seemed much less anxious and fearful at the end of the four weeks. The counselor continued to check in periodically with Chris and Chris's parents throughout the rest of the school year.

In the fall of the fourth grade, Chris saw the counselor primarily thorough classroom guidance. In the spring, the counselor and several teachers nominated Chris to participate in counselor-led training as a peer helper. As Chris had moved through elementary school, social interest and social skills had become one of Chris's most evident strengths. Chris seemed a very good candidate for being a kindergarten buddy. Chris's parents agreed to Chris's participation in the training, and Chris eagerly entered into training sessions. The training occurred the last month of the fourth grade so the helpers could assume their responsibilities when they began fifth grade.

As a fifth grader, Chris enjoyed being a peer buddy to a kindergarten child. Chris was responsible, never missing a peer session. Chris demonstrated caring and gave much encouragement when playing with the kindergarten buddy. Chris met regularly with the counselor and other peer helpers for feedback sessions and reviews of helping skills. During the fifth grade, Chris also participated in classroom guidance lessons led by the counselor to help students prepare to enter middle school. Toward the close of the school year, the elementary school counselor coordinated with the special education teacher an outing for Chris and other students with special needs to visit the middle school and to be introduced to the school staff, including the middle school counselor.

Editors' Note:

   Palmer, Deck, and Brotherton provided unique and caring examples of the school counselor's role in interdisciplinary service provision. One area not considered, however, is assisting with children with disabilities when they are teased or rejected by others. Rude stares, teasing and rejection may not be viewed as abuse, but the results of these behaviors is abusive. The counselor, as well as teachers and other school personnel should assist the student with developing strategies to understand and cope with the rude, though often unintentional, actions of others.

   Dr. Schulz notes that although Billy is an adult, she and he still deal with long, hard stares. She states that this is usually the result of ignorance. Furthermore, she suggests that as students who are typical have common experiences with students with disabilities, the staring ceases. Dr. Schulz finds that teasing and rejection are less obvious than staring and more difficult to deal with. Sometimes, as referred to in another chapter, students with disabilities need to develop social skills to reduce the probability that they will be targets of teasing and rejection. Likewise, typical students need awareness and understanding of the problems their actions can impose.

REFERENCES

Borders, L. D., & Drury, S. M. (1992). Comprehensive school counseling programs: A review for policy makers and practitioners. *Journal of Counseling and Development, 70,* 487-498.

Greer, B. B., Greer, J. G., & Woody, D. E. (1995). The inclusion movement and its impact on counselors. *The School Counselor, 43,* 124-132.

Myrick, R. D., & Dixon, R. W. (1985). Changing student attitudes and behavior through group counseling. *The School Counselor, 32,* 325-330.

Omizo, M. M., & Omizo, S. A. (1987). Group counseling with children of divorce: New findings. *Elementary School Guidance and Counseling, 22,* 46-52.

Paisley, P.O., & Hubbard, G.T. (1989). School counseling: State officials' perceptions of certification and employment trends. *Counselor Education and Supervision, 29*, 60-70.

Schmidt, J.J. (1996). *Counseling in schools* (2nd ed.) Boston: Allyn and Bacon.

Sylwester, R. (1995). *A celebration of neurons: An educators' guide to the human brain.* Alexandria, VA: Association for Supervision and Curriculum Development.

Chapter 15

SOCIAL WORK

NANCY P. KROPF AND KEVIN L. DEWEAVER

When the American version of social work was developing in the late 1800s, there was a major focus on children and families but not on people with disabilities. Over time, in the twentieth century, social work began to make contributions in the disability field. In the 1960s, social workers entered the field of mental retardation in significant numbers and delivered services to a group of people who had been ignored for many years. During the 1970s, social work broadened its horizons with the developmental disability concept and significantly contributed to the deinstitutionalization movement (DeWeaver, 1983). Throughout the 1980s and 1990s, social work has supported the broadening of the disability concept and the inclusion of more people who need various types of social services.

Social workers provide services in a wide range of settings found throughout the disabilities field. When many people think of disabilities and social work, they think of state institutions. Today this perception is changing, as nearly 40 percent of these institutions have been closed since 1960 (Lakin, Prouty, Anderson, & Sandlin, 1997). Currently social workers in this field practice in the following settings: community-based residences (formerly called group homes), various medical settings (public and private), local service boards, state departments, and a variety of schools. Additionally, social workers may deliver services to people with disabilities who are in other service networks (e.g., mental health, corrections).

MAJOR ROLES AND RESPONSIBILITIES SOCIAL WORK

The roles and responsibilities of social workers have been, and continue to be, varied and broad in nature. In discussing past contributions of social workers in the field of developmental disabilities, Horejsi (1979) noted the following typical tasks: the provision of individual and group counseling (e.g., to children with mental retardation, their parents, and their siblings); the provision of social histories as part of the diagnostic process; the development of community residences, including foster homes; the development of protective services and advocacy services; the provision of case management services in a service network; and community organization and social planning activities. More recently further emphasis is being placed on supportive counseling and the role of advocacy which is congruent with Hanley and Parkinson's (1994) call for social workers to develop and implement more family support and home care programs.

Social workers often provide services to children with disabilities in the school setting due to the passage of P.L. 94-142 in 1975. Besides the traditional direct service activities of a clinical social worker, school social workers may have to perform additional duties such as coordinating Individualized Educational Program conferences, promoting or developing self-help groups that provide support systems to the families of children with disabilities, serving as trained mediators in service contract negotiations, and leading parent groups focused on education around a certain issue or information about service delivery.

As described, the roles that social workers perform are many and varied. While many are direct service oriented, others relate to working with professionals and on behalf of children with disabilities and their families. Kaufman, DeWeaver, and Glicken (1989) have pointed out the importance of six basic roles:

1. outreach worker role—identifies and assesses clients;
2. advocate role—protects and promotes clients' rights;
3. teacher role—provides information at a variety of levels (e.g., individual, community);
4. therapist role—provides counseling and therapy to improve social functioning;
5. enabler/facilitator role—aids clients to recognize their strengths and seeks to help clients to help themselves; and
6. broker/coordinator role—links clients to needed services as well as providing the necessary follow-up activities to see that the clients are receiving what they need.

The characteristic that distinguishes social work from other disciplines can be given in one word: *breadth,* which can be seen in the variety of settings discussed above. Another way to see the diversity in social work practice is by viewing the different career paths that social workers can take. While the direct service social worker is very familiar to most people in this field, social workers in areas such as administration, program evaluation, policy analysis, and research are not well known but serve critical functions. A final distinguishing characteristic of social work is its focus, which has been described best as the person-in-environment framework. Essentially a social worker's focus is not on the individual totally or even the circumstances, but rather on the *interactions* that take place with the unique client and his or her environment. This is a very effective, unique approach that tends to individualize and personalize the professional relationship. This personalization is usually needed when working with children with disabilities and their families who may often have gotten the "red tape" approach in the past.

CONTRIBUTIONS OF SOCIAL WORK TO INTERDISCIPLINARY PRACTICE

There are four models of team practice that are generally observed: intradisciplinary, transdisciplinary, multidisciplinary, and interdisciplinary (Rokusek, 1995). The latter model, which is also referred to as the interprofessional team, has gained popularity over the last two decades and is characterized "where each member is viewed as an equal in all decision-making and consensus-building" (Rokusek, 1995, p. 5).

As might be expected, social workers contribute to interdisciplinary practice by performing a variety of activities, which may or may not be labeled case management. One major contribution is the psychosocial assessment of children with disabilities and their families. There has been a movement away from the medical model and toward a strengths perspective, which emphasizes the uniqueness of the family and the individual. In this emerging model, labels must be used carefully if at all. Standardized instruments, such as the revised 52-item Questionnaire on Resources and Stress, are available to aid the social worker in family assessment (Levy, 1995). It is important that the assessment contain information about what is being requested and the objectives of the client and his or her family. From an accurate assessment and problem identification, a social worker could "involve problem solving and negotiation to look for new solutions or recommendations, acting as an educator or liaison to obtain necessary training for family members, or helping team members and family see the perspectives of one another and communicate with one another" (Levy, 1995, p. 195).

From the interdisciplinary assessment and group process, a plan (e.g., an Individualized Education Program) is negotiated and then must be implemented. The implementation phase is often conceptualized in a frame of reference where the social worker can be assigned as the case manager. As there has been confusion about this term, a simple definition is as follows: "Case management is a set of logical steps and a process of interaction within a service network which assures that a client receives needed services in a supportive, effective, efficient, and cost-effective manner" (Weil & Karls, 1985, p. 2). Case management in the developmental disability field uses a comprehensive model that is very service intensive and time consuming, thus the number of clients must be held down to a reasonable number (e.g., 20-25) for effective service and necessary follow-up to be done.

Case management has been adopted by the National Association of Social Workers (1992), who revised the four standards for case management that follow:

- *Standard one. Enhancing Self-Determinism.* It is the responsibility of the social work case manager to assure that clients are involved in the development and implementation of their own care plans to the greatest possible extent;
- *Standard two. Primacy of Client's Interests.* The social work case manager should serve clients with the maximum application of professional skill and weigh carefully organizational goals in relation to the client's needs;
- *Standard three. Confidentiality and Privacy.* As case manager, the social worker should work with other professions and other agency staff in a manner which protects the individual's rights to privacy and assures appropriate confidentiality when information is released to others; and
- *Standard four. Relationship with Colleagues.* As case manager, the social worker should treat colleagues with courtesy and respect and strive to enhance interprofessional cooperation on behalf of the client.

Historically the last standard may be the most difficult to achieve. In discussing special educators and social workers, Lynch (1981) stated, "all too often neither discipline has understood the other's role or function ... and each discipline has retreated and hidden behind a wall of jargon, misunderstanding, and mistrust" (p. 163). While things have improved greatly today, the potential for retreating to the unfavorable conditions of the past must be guarded against. The elements of mutual respect and open communication are essential for effective, cooperative interdisciplinary practice. Hence, Lynch (1981) has suggested the following guidelines by which to practice:

1. I will learn your language and teach you mine,
2. I will ask for your perceptions and feedback, not for praise or affirmation, but to learn more of what you know and to challenge my own timeworn positions,
3. I will share my professional strengths and my weakness with you so that we can both grow,

4. I will not withhold "disciplinary secrets" from you, or cling tenaciously to my turf; but I will tell you when I am feeling invaded and expect you to do the same; and

5. I will confront you, challenge you, listen to you, and learn from you. I will expect you to do the same with me. (p. 176)

The above guidelines would make for ideal collaborative teamwork. In reality it may be an ideal to strive for rather expect. Recent changes, such as managed care, have aided in making "turf guarding" an issue again. Obviously, these disputes between disciplines do nothing to aid the child with a disability or his/her family. However, as barriers to good practice, they must first be acknowledged before they can be resolved.

Finally, it must be noted that a social worker's role on a team or as a case manager will vary if he or she is practicing in a rural area. Given limited resources in such areas, the social worker can expect more client contact and less referral to other professionals (DeWeaver & Johnson, 1983). The role of resource creator may also be added as the continuum of rurality increases in their job. Hence, a good generalist background is suggested for social workers who may deliver disability services in rural areas.

ROLES PARENTS PLAY IN OPTIMAL INTERDISCIPLINARY SERVICE PROVISION OF SOCIAL WORK

Previously, parents and formal service providers, including social workers, did not work collaboratively on service goals of a child with a developmental disability. In fact, parents and professionals may have been at odds, working on different goals for the same child. Kropf (1997) discusses the adversarial relationship that existed between previous cohorts of parents and service providers. Older parents may still mistrust social workers, physicians, or other professionals because of negative experiences that they faced when their child was young. Examples include physicians who told parents that their only option was to institutionalize a child, or social workers who argued with parents about best practices for raising a child with a disability. The negative encounters can have lasting impact on parents' impressions of service professionals.

Thankfully, much has changed in developmental disability services since the 1940s and 1950s. The current model of service stresses collaboration between a family and the social work professional. The role of the social worker is to individualize the particular family's resources, desires, and needs by way of understanding the current situation of the family, and working with the family to avoid unexpected or crisis situations at future points. An example of this goal would be to have a family begin to use respite care services early in life. This provides parents with the opportunity to focus on other things, such as taking a trip away as a couple or spending time with other children in the family. The child with a disability, in turn, learns how to be away from the family and builds levels of self-sufficiency and independence.

Parents have important roles to play in working with the social worker on an interdisciplinary team. One role is an *informant*, which is helping the social worker understand how the family functions including points of stress and reward in raising a child with a disability. A second role is to be a *clarifier*, which is to enable the social worker to "make sense" of why a family acts in a particular way or has a certain priority. For example, behavior that may look problematic on the surface may have a place or function in a particular family. A third role is that of an *active agent*, that is, working with the social worker and the rest of the team to put a plan into action for the child with disabilities. Each of these roles will be addressed, and case examples of each are provided.

Informant

Although a team of service providers can learn about a child's behavior, the real "experts" about the child are the parents and other family members. Their input is important to the social worker and interdisciplinary team. Even if the social worker spends time in the child's classroom or makes home visits, the parent is with the son or daughter in more situations than any professional can possibly be. This expertise is important for the team to put together a service plan for the child and family.

There are several different types of information that a parent can provide. One is how the child functions in different situations. Some of this information may be gathered by talking with the child himself or herself, or observing him/her in various situations. However, parents may have insight that is not shared by any other source. For example, some children may have difficulty with new situations. A child may do fine in the household or in the classroom, but may have behavioral outbursts during times when the family travels, goes on outings, or is away from familiar surroundings. Another source of information is about the relationships between other family members and the child. A child may relate well to certain family members, but may have problems with others. For example, a mother may share her perception that an older sister is impatient with a younger child who has a disability. That insight should be followed up by the social worker to assess whether the sister might benefit from some program to help her with some of the issues of having a sibling with a disability.

In addition to current information, parents should also be involved in examining future needs of the family. While things may be going well at one point in time, families continue to face changes across the life span that impact the ability to provide care. For example, one of the authors of this chapter worked with a family who was raising a child with cerebral palsy. The family functioned well when the child was young; however, when the child entered the teen years the mother started to experience health problems as a result of the continued transferring and lifting that was necessary. This information prompted the interdisciplinary team to explore several options including structural changes in the household, in-home support services, and education for the parents about healthier ways to complete lifts and transfers.

Clarifier

Another role that parents can play is to help in clarifying expectations, goals, and desires of the family. Many different characteristics can impact on how a particular family functions including past ways of operating, and cultural or religious values that are important to the family. Even the behavior that may seem maladaptive on the surface may have an important outcome in the family. In sharing this information with the social worker and the rest of the team, the parents help the service providers in structuring plans of action that are consistent with what the family holds as important.

One important area is the family's cultural or religious beliefs. Many research studies suggest that families who are members of ethnic minorities may not have the same needs or service goals as Caucasian families (Helter, Markwardt, Rowitz, & Farber, 1994; Rogers-Dulan & Blacher, 1995). This is unfortunate, since most research about what families need or desire includes few persons who are from various racial/ethnic groups. In social work education curriculum, multicultural issues are explored and discussed. However, this information must be understood within the context of a particular family. For example, Jewish parents might be adamant that a son with mental retardation participate in classes to prepare for his bar mitzvah. Culturally, this celebration is one of achieving an adult status within the faith. If the child is able to participate in instruction, this would be a cause for celebration for the child and family. However, if the child does not have the skills to complete this process, the social worker should be available to help the family work through any feelings of loss, disappointment, or frustration that might be experienced.

Active Agent

In most situations, parents have a pivotal role in moving a service plan into an action plan with the child. This may include being in situations that seem harsh or difficult. Sometimes, interdisciplinary teams are involved in creating behavior modification plans for children who have maladaptive behaviors. An important aspect is to provide consistency in these plans across settings. If the targeted behavior is to reduce tantrums of a child, it is important that the plan be implemented in all settings that tantrums exist. A behavior plan might include rewarding a child when she or he remains on task and ignoring behavioral outbursts. The theory is that any attention will reinforce behavior, even if the attention is negative (e.g., shouting at child, pleading with child to stop crying). Some parents might find this approach difficult and revert back to previous ways of stopping a child's tantrum such as offering toys or candy as a diversion. While this might quiet the child in the short term, it does nothing to change the behavior. In this instance, it is important that the parents act as active agents in adhering to the goals of the service plan.

In addition to promoting consistency in a service plan, parents may need to participate in evaluating the outcomes of a particular course of action. One way that determinations are made about whether a plan of action is working is to chart or monitor progress. Parents may be asked to participate in gathering this information. Here is an example of how parents would provide information to the team about progress with intervention. In the previous example of an older sibling who was impatient with a younger brother or sister with a disability, the social worker may invite the teen to participate in a group specifically for siblings. These groups provide a time for children in the family to discuss the stresses and rewards of having a brother or sister with a disability. The intended outcome is to process their feelings with others in the same situation, and learn from one another about ways to handle some of the stress that they experience. Parents can provide information about how the teen interacts with the younger child - are there less arguments, is the teen more patient? Those outcomes would suggest that the intervention, the support group, is having the intended impact on the teen.

PARENT QUESTIONS REGARDING THE ROLE OF THE SOCIAL WORKER

As in the other chapters of the text, parents were invited to provide questions for each discipline. For social work, parents seemed most interested in how to be sure that the intervention programs are quality ones for their child and how to access needed services. Parents also wanted to know more about how a child's disability may impact on other members of their family. A few of the questions posed by parents are presented in the following section.

I want the best for my child. How can I make certain that his intervention programs are challenging, positive, and have integrity and vision?

The parent(s) who raised this question should be commended for the attention to quality programs for the child. The person who posed this question is concerned that the child's program provide his or her son/daughter with an opportunity for growth and stimulation. From a social work perspective, this attitude conveys a parent who is interested in the child's progress and ready to be part of a team that can help a child accomplish his or her goals!

The first, and most basic, recommendation is to maintain continued involvement with the interdisciplinary team. As stated earlier in this chapter, parents have the greatest expertise about their child and make significant contributions. Sometimes it might feel overwhelming to have to attend yet another meeting at the school, or go through an intake session at the community service board. However, persistence does bring rewards. It is frustrating for the social worker to work on a quality service plan with a parent, and then have a family become disinterested or disengaged from the process. Quality programs demand investments of time, energy, and commitment from service professionals and parents alike. As social workers, the authors encourage the parent to remain active and continue to participate in this process!

Another role for parents is to become self-educated about options that are possibilities for the child. Parents can bring a sense of creativity to the team process, and help the professionals break away from the usual way of thinking about service provision. About ten years ago, a family moved to the community where the authors of this chapter work. Their teen age son has developmental and physical disabilities and was getting near the age of adulthood. After the parents discussed options with the local community service agency, they decided that a standard residential placement, such as a group home, would not work for their son. Instead, the family joined with others in the community who were having similar frustrations with the lack of options for their adult children. By researching programs in other states, they started a nonprofit service program to allow people with disabilities to rent or purchase homes and receive support services in their own households. This is a remarkable change from the previous practice of having people with disabilities move to congregate living facilities such as group homes, supported living arrangements or nursing homes. This initiative was started by parents who became self-educated about other options, and worked to bring them to their community.

On a similar note, parents can assess intervention programs and plans by networking with other parents who face similar issues. One way is to become involved in parent groups in the local community which may be formed through the school district, community service boards, churches/synagogues, or other organizations. These forums provide parents with an opportunity to share experiences with other parents and to be able to assess whether a child's program could be made more comprehensive, challenging, or rewarding. In addition to personal contact, parents are able to network with others throughout the world by electronic means. For parents who have problems finding time to attend face-to-face meetings, the use of a computer allows them to link with others. There are many organizations that have a home page on the World Wide Web as well as electronic discussion groups where parents can share ideas and views.

A part of the question that was posed introduced an interesting element; does the program have vision and is it challenging? This aspect makes an important assumption that parents need to consider, that is, what does the future hold for my child? As children without disabilities begin to develop and gain greater independence, parents often begin to think about the future of a son or daughter. Certain choices may help steer a child into a certain direction, for example, a mother who enrolls a young daughter in an after school dance or musical program to foster creative talent. However, there may not be a similar process or option when the child has a disability. In fact, one of the common questions that parents ask social workers is, "what does the future hold for my son or daughter with a disability?" As parents begin to plan for their child's future, these thoughts need to be shared with service providers so plans can include appropriate goals. For example, a child who is terrified of being apart from a parent would have a difficult time going to camp. However, the parents may want to use a camp experience as a respite for them and also as a way to help their son or daughter build skills toward independence. The social worker on the team can be helpful in working with parents to think about the future of their child, and ways to construct plans to help the child develop and grow in those areas.

Do you have suggestions or resources to help me help my other children deal with their sister's disability?

The question raised by this parent is one that is frequently posed to social workers. Often, parents may feel that the attention, time, and effort that is expended on a child with a disability may make other children in the family feel left out or unimportant. Due to the time and financial expenses of caregiving, there may also be fewer opportunities to do things that other families do together. One of the authors of this chapter was a social worker in a community mental health center in Michigan, which is a state that provides a family support subsidy. A family who were clients of the agency had a child with severe mental retardation, cerebral palsy, and other medical problems. This family had extensive out-of-pocket expenses for their son who took several medications, was hospitalized frequently, and needed specialized equipment. When the family qualified for the subsidy, they used their monthly payments to purchase a specialized van, which could transport their son in his wheelchair. Due to his extensive disabilities, he was most comfortable remaining in his chair during trips instead of sitting in the car seat. The new van allowed the family to do something that they had never done together before—take a family vacation. They packed up their van and went to an amusement park where the other children in the family took turns pushing their brother's wheelchair around the park, feeding him cotton candy, and having a great time. The point is, that without additional resources, this family might never had done what most families do—take a vacation together and enjoy each other's company. Social workers can assist families in identifying resources and strategies that allow families to do things together and promote a sense of family unity.

Many brothers and sisters of children with disabilities can benefit from being involved in a support group with children from other families. These groups provide siblings with an opportunity to share their experiences of having a brother or sister with a disability. In these support groups, brothers and sisters can discuss both the frustrations and rewards of being with their sibling. Some of the common stresses experienced are having to babysit more than their friends, wondering how to handle situations involving their brother or sister with their peers, and fearing that they will have to have their brother or sister live with them when they are adults. However, brothers and sisters also report benefits in their relationship with their sibling. Positive aspects of the relationship include being more patient and tolerant, and learning how to become more responsible. These issues can be topics of conversation in a group for older children and teenagers. Discussing both stresses and rewards helps put their relationship with their brother and sister into a more rounded perspective.

The issue of future care is an important one for families and does have implications for relationships between siblings. Research on family planning for the future of a child with a disability suggests that many parents do not have any plans at the point where they can no longer provide care (Freedman, Krauss, & Seltzer, 1997; Kaufman, Adams, & Campbell, 1991). The assumption of some parents is that a brother or sister will become the primary care provider after they become ill or die. Some siblings are willing and have the resources to become the caregiver. In other families, however, this expectation is unrealistic or unfeasible. For a number of reasons, siblings can be a valuable resource across the life span for their brother or sister with a disability. However, parents should begin future care plans before problems occur such as a parental illness or death. This can alleviate fears and anxieties by siblings who feel trapped into assuming primary care of their brother or sister, and offer time to explore other options prior to a crisis. Social workers can assist with future care planning and work with the family to identify and evaluate various options that are available.

Dr. Schulz's Response:

The authors' response dealing with relationships among siblings is excellent. As parents, we need to spend time with all our children, although the child with a disability may require more time. I was startled when my youngest child, as a teenager, said to me, "You know, I never got to be the baby."

My three children, siblings of Billy, acknowledge the positive effects he has had on their lives. However, only one of them has expressed the wish to be responsible for him in the event of my death. We cannot assume that our children will accept this responsibility, nor should we expect them to. Another consideration in this scenario is the spouse of the sibling, a person who did not grow up with a child who has a disability.

With the help of social workers and others involved with your child, a number of alternatives can be explored to help plan for your child's future. The entire family should be involved in discussing these alternatives and in developing the appropriate plan, keeping in mind that the plan may, and probably will, change with changes in the status of the family and with the addition of alternatives in the community.

The social worker involved in my child's evaluation took a long and intimate family history. At times, I felt a little uncomfortable. What is the purpose of this in the evaluation process, and how can it be less intrusive?

One of the cardinal principles of social work is to individualize clients' or families' situations as a way to understand the particular problems that they are experiencing, their resources and coping styles, and ways to intervene in situations. In an interdisciplinary team, the social worker is commonly assigned the task of conducting a psychosocial history. This process involves learning about the child's and family's history and how events (even those that seem distant and unrelated to the current situation) may have an impact on the current family situation. For example, parents may be asked questions about their relationship and how raising a child with a disability has altered their marriage. One part of this question may include their sexual relationship. This may be embarrassing for the parents to discuss, yet the answer provides the social worker with valuable information about how the mother and father relate to one another. After the birth of any child, all parents can expect to lose some degree of romance, intimacy, and spontaneity in their relationship. Due to the demands of raising a child with a disability, parents can experience stress on their marriage which decreases the satisfaction with intimate aspects of their relationship. If parents report this to a social worker, one part of a service plan may be a referral to a marriage counselor for the parents to work on some relationship issues.

In social work education programs, a tremendous amount of classroom and internship time is spent on helping students develop into sensitive and effective professionals. An analogy with the medical field may help make this point. Few women enjoy going to their annual physical examination with their gynecologist. During this process it is natural to feel uncomfortable, anxious, uneasy, and vulnerable. However, it is necessary because only through the exam procedure does the physician gather the right type of information to help the patient become or remain healthy. The goal of the physician is to gather data—it is not to make value judgments about the patient. Social workers are professionals who have been trained to gather information from clients as a way of putting together a picture of the individual's and family's functioning. Questions, even ones that seem intrusive, may have an important place in determining problems or strengths of the family. Like the physician, the social worker does not engage in an evaluation with clients to judge them, but as a way to gather information to construct a service plan that can truly help a family.

As a parent, it is your right to understand why a particular line of questioning is being pursued by a social worker. If questions are being posed that seem unreasonable or unconnected to your family situation, feel free to ask! One approach is to say to the social worker, "The questions that you are asking are very personal ones and make me feel uncomfortable answering. Will you explain to me why these questions are included in this evaluation? Also, since the answers are private to my family, how will my answers be used? And who else will have access to this information?" The answer to these questions may help you feel more comfortable that the information that you provide is relevant and confidential, and will not be shared with inappropriate sources. If you still are uncomfortable, ask if this information is required for the services you are requesting. If it is not, do not answer items that are problematic for you. After the social worker provides you with the response, you could say something like this, "Thank you for taking time to explain why these questions are included. However, I still feel uncomfortable providing the answers as the topics are private and personal to me. My preference is to skip over these questions unless it will negatively impact the services that my child can receive."

CASE EXAMPLE

Annie is an eight-year-old child whose family was requesting services through a community mental health center that offered services to people with developmental disabilities. Annie has multiple impairments including cerebral palsy, mental retardation, asthma, a heart murmur, and suffers from chronic respiratory infections. She was brought to the intake evaluation by her mother, who is not employed outside the home. The primary service that the parents requested was respite care as the family had been unable to locate anyone who could provide temporary breaks in caregiving.

The procedure for an intake was to have the social worker conduct a psychosocial assessment with the mother and Annie. As part of this process, the person with a disability is encouraged to participate to the greatest degree possible. Annie is functionally nonverbal, but she was included in the intake, which provided the social worker with an opportunity to evaluate her social skills. The psychosocial assessment takes about 45 minutes on average to complete and includes questions related to the child's developmental history, functional level, information about the parents and other family members, and social support systems of the family. Sometimes, the parent may be asked to provide consent to request records from other agencies such as the child's school or physician.

After the intake is complete, the social worker constructs an intake evaluation report to share with the interdisciplinary team at the weekly staffing session. The purpose of the staffing is to share information about the new client and decide who will be the primary staff member to work with the family. Usually, that decision is determined by the type of service request that the family has made. In Annie's situation, the social worker was assigned as the primary person to work with the family and the social worker assumed the role as *case manager.* As case manager, the social worker will work with the team in constructing a service plan, take responsibility for coordinating the various aspects of the plan, and act as the liaison with other agencies such as Annie's school. In addition, the case manager will periodically bring up Annie's case information to review at the interdisciplinary team meeting. The agency mandates that a review be done once a year, or at a more frequent interval if there is a dramatic change in the family's or Annie's situation. The social worker provided a brief summary of Annie's situation that included the following information.

Client and Family Functioning

Annie is an eight-year-old girl who has cerebral palsy, mental retardation, respiratory and heart conditions. Annie is nonverbal, uses a wheelchair, has limited gross motor skills and no fine motor skills. She is enrolled in a self-contained special education class for children with physical and developmental disabilities. Her family includes a mother who is not employed outside the home, father who works as a supervisor in a manufacturing plant, and two older sisters. Her grandparents and other extended family live out of state.

Socially, Annie is a gregarious child. She enjoys her school program and gets along well with her teacher and other children in the class. She and her mother share a warm and positive relationship, and Annie will coo and smile when her mother talks. There was limited information presented about Annie's father. He has a job that is very demanding and he often works overtime hours. The mother described him as a "workaholic" and states that he rarely is around the house on weekends or evenings. Annie gets along well with her older sister, Jean, who is 15. However, her 12-year-old sister, Melissa, has become a problem for the parents and has started acting out in school and in the household. Recently, this sister was suspended from school for starting a fire in the bathroom. The mother states that this is one of the problems that the family is facing. The mother is finding it difficult to manage the parenting demands of Annie, who is totally dependent in all areas of functioning, in addition to trying to handle Melissa. Since the father is rarely at home, the responsibility falls to the mother and sometimes to Jean.

In addition, some additional historical information was gathered that provides a deeper understanding of current functioning. Annie was the product of a normal pregnancy, although the parents had not planned for a third child. During the birth process, there were medical complications which resulted in Annie's developmental and medical conditions. The parents were notified immediately after birth that there were complications. Annie stayed in the hospital neonatal ICU for several weeks. She has been hospitalized about seven times since birth.

The news about Annie's medical problems was difficult for the family. As the mother states, "My husband did not want to believe that Annie's condition would be permanent. Throughout the first two years of her life, he kept stating that we would find a doctor who could cure her of these problems." The family went to several physicians, all of whom confirmed that Annie would have several developmental disabilities. Through her faith and support from her own parents, the mother has come to accept Annie and her disabilities. However, she states that her husband interacts with his daughter as little as possible. In fact, his relationship with the other girls has also changed as he no longer spends time with them as he did previously. He states that he has to be at work more hours to be able to pay for the costs associated with Annie's condition. This situation leaves him little time to spend with the family.

Social Support

The family moved from their home state when Annie was two so the father could accept a job promotion at the plant. Before they moved, the mother was employed part-time in a publishing firm. The maternal grandparents lived very close, and the grandmother would provide care for Annie while the mother was at work. With the relocation, the family moved to a community where they did not know anyone. The family made some friends through the church, but the family does not feel comfortable asking for assistance in providing supervision for Annie. Although her care is not complicated, it does involve transferring, lifting, and toileting.

For the most part, the parents have few social outlets. The father works an average of 60 to 70 hours in a typical week. This schedule provides extra money for the family, but keeps him from being involved in the household on any regular basis. The mother reports that she is socially isolated. She misses her work, as she enjoyed her previous employment and being connected to others in the workplace. Rarely do the parents spent time together as a couple; the mother reported that she and her husband have not done anything alone since they relocated.

Jean and Melissa have made friends through their school. In addition, Jean is athletic and joined the volleyball and track teams at her school. The mother laments that she has not been able to attend Jean's matches since it is difficult to transport Annie to the games. She states that she used to be athletic herself, and wishes that she could relive some of the excitement through Jean's participation in sports. On the other hand, Melissa has never been interested in extracurricular activities. A shy child, she recently became more involved with new friends when she entered middle school. It was at that point that Melissa began to experience greater problems in school and at home. She has been caught skipping classes, she once was brought home for shoplifting, and recently was suspended for two weeks for setting a fire in the school bathroom. The mother describes Melissa as "angry" and the tension between Melissa and her father has escalated since her school suspension. As the mother put it, "Melissa used to idolize Jean, but now she doesn't want to have anything to do with anyone in the family." Annie and Jean are close, but Melissa and Annie are not.

Requests for Service

The mother's original request was for respite care for the family. She perceives that respite would allow her to spend time with her husband, and have the family do some things together, like see Jean compete. It is the mother's impression that this may resolve some of the problems with Melissa.

As part of the intake, the social worker provided information about other services that are available in the agency, or resources in the community. One of those that interested the mother was the family support groups that are offered through the agency. These groups allow parents to come together and discuss issues of raising a child with a disability. These groups are cofacilitated by the psychologist and social worker from the interdisciplinary team. Although the mother was interested, she did not believe that her husband would attend as "he does not like sharing his business with people outside the family." In conjunction with the group, respite care is provided by paraprofessional staff at the agency so families do not have to be concerned with finding substitute care to attend. The mother was also excited that Annie would have the chance to be around other children, as she enjoys being in social situations.

Recommendations of the Interdisciplinary Team

Based upon the psychosocial summary provided by the social worker, the interdisciplinary team made the following recommendations.

These would be followed up with the social worker who was serving as the case manager of the team. The team requested that the case be presented again after six months to determine whether any changes had taken place as a result of the recommendations with the family.

Provide Agency-based Respite Care Services to the Family

The agency can provide paraprofessional respite care in the family home a maximum of two times per month. The family would coordinate the dates and times with the social worker, who would match a respite provider with the family.

Supplement formal respite services with informal respite sources. Due to the limitations in the agency respite services, the social worker will work with the family to identify other sources of respite care. One will be with members of the family's church congregation. The agency could be helpful in working out ways to secure additional respite providers. The following possibilities were posed by the team:

- Social worker assist mother in discussing situation with pastor of the church to find out if there is way of getting members of the congregation to volunteer as providers.
- Although Annie's care is not complicated, there are certain skills involved. If volunteers are secured through the church, the nurse on the team would co-lead a training session with the social worker in the fam-

ily's home. During this time, volunteers would learn how to do transfers and lifts with Annie.

Support the Mother in Joining the Parent Group

The team supported the mother's desire to join the parent group. This connection can have many benefits for her, even if her husband chooses not to attend. It will provide her with the option of increasing her own social network through associations with the other parents in the group. In addition, she can learn from other parents about some of the struggles that she faces in her own family—lack of involvement from the father, tension with Melissa, for example.

Explore Family Counseling

The team discussed the dynamics of this family at length. There are some important issues going on that could be helped through work with a family counselor at the agency. Some of the dynamics that were noted by the team include the father's lack of participation in the household and the distance between him, his daughters, and his wife. In addition, Melissa's maladaptive behaviors in school and how these may be related to being a "lost child," are not receiving attention by excelling (like Jean) or needing extensive supports (like Annie).

The psychologist recommended meeting with the family, if they agreed, to explain about the family counseling resources that were available at the agency. While no sibling group exists at the present time, the team is starting to consider forming one.

Referral to Social Activities for Annie

In addition to these services for the family, the team also recommended that the social worker explore other activities that are available for Annie. Besides her classroom, she has limited interaction with other children and her primary relationship is with her mother and older sister. Unfortunately, limited options for recreation activities are available for people with disabilities. However, the social worker would explore this issue further.

This example demonstrates several points about interdisciplinary team approaches to working with children who have disabilities. One is that needs within the family are also explored, such as the dynamics of the family and relationships between parents and other children. Another aspect is that, based upon a comprehensive intake evaluation, the team was able to make recommendations that were beyond the initial service request of the client. While the social worker was assigned as the case manager for Annie, the recommendations in the service plan brought in the expertise of other professionals including the nurse and psychologist. All of these factors promote a comprehensive way to serve people with disabilities and their families.

Editor's Note:

Kropf and DeWeaver have done an excellent job of delineating the roles and responsibilities of social workers and families in interdisciplinary contexts. One important issue is confidentiality. Dr. Schulz notes that privacy is difficult to maintain. She recently encountered a classroom teacher who, in describing her difficult year in a social situation, went into great detail about the characteristics, family background, and behavior of a child who had severe behavior disorders. This conversation clearly abused this child's rights to confidentiality. We think that all of us can learn a lesson from social work's strong commitment to confidentiality.

REFERENCES

DeWeaver, K.L. (1983). Deinstitutionalization of the developmentally disabled. *Social Work, 28,* 435-439.

DeWeaver, K. L., & Johnson, P. J. (1983). Case management in rural areas for the developmentally disabled. *Human Services in the Rural Environment, 8* (4), 23-31.

Freedman, R. I., Krauss, M. W., & Seltzer, M. M. (1997). Aging parents' residential plans for adult children with mental retardation. *Mental Retardation, 35,* 114-123.

Hanley, B., & Parkinson, C. B. (1994). Position paper on social work values: Practice with individuals who have developmental disabilities. *Mental Retardation, 32,* 426-431.

Helter, T., Markwardt, R., Rowitz, L., & Farber, B. (1994). Adaptation of Hispanic families to a member with mental retardation. *American Journal on Mental Retardation, 99,* 289300.

Horejsi, C. R. (1979). Developmental disabilities: Opportunities for social workers. *Social Work, 24,* 40-43.

Kaufman, A. V., Adams, J. P., & Campbell, V. A. (1991). Permanency planning by older parents who care for adult children with mental retardation. *Mental Retardation, 29,* 293-300.

Kaufman, A. V., DeWeaver, K. L., & Glicken, M. (1989). The mentally retarded aged: Implications for social work practice. *Journal of Gerontological Social Work, 14,* 93-110.

Kropf, N. P. (1997). Older parents of adults with developmental disabilities: Practice issues and service needs. *Journal of Family Psychotherapy, 8,* 35-52.

Lakin, K. C., Prouty, B., Anderson, L., & Sandlin, J. (1997). Nearly 40% of state institutions have been closed. *Mental Retardation, 35,* 65.

Levy, J. M. (1995). Social Work. In B. A. Thyer & N. P. Kropf (Eds.), *Developmental disabilities: A handbook for interdisciplinary practice* (pp. 188-201). Cambridge, MA: Brookline.

Lynch, E. W. (1981). The social worker as part of an interdisciplinary team. In M. U. Dickerson, *Social work practice with the mentally retarded* (pp. 162-176). New York: Free Press.

National Association of Social Workers. (1992). NASW standards for social work case management. Washington, DC: Author.

Rogers-Dulan, J., & Blacher, J. (1995). African American families, religion, and disability: A conceptual framework. *Mental Retardation, 33*, 226-238.

Rokusek, C. (1995). An introduction to the concept of interdisciplinary practice. In B. A. Thyer & N. P. Kropf (Eds.), *Developmental disabilities: A handbook for interdisciplinary practice* (pp. 1-12). Cambridge, MA: Brookline.

Weil, M., & Karls, J. M. (1985). Historical origins and recent developments. In M. Weils, J. M. Karls, & Associates (Eds.), *Case management in human service practice* (pp. 1-10). San Francisco: Jossey-Bass.

Chapter 16

FUTURE DIRECTIONS FOR PARENTS AND PROFESSIONALS IN INTERDISCIPLINARY SERVICE DELIVERY

BILLY T. OGLETREE, JANE B. SCHULZ AND MARTIN A. FISCHER

It is our hope that the reader of this book has gained a broad understanding of interdisciplinary practice from the perspectives of professionals who participate in team-based services for children with disabilities and their families. We would like to think that the dialogue between chapter authors, parents, and the editors has furthered the reader's knowledge in terms of identifying and addressing issues relevant to today's team.

This final chapter is an attempt to focus the reader on what we believe will be central practice issues for tomorrow's interdisciplinary team. First, Dr. Ogletree discusses two themes that resonate throughout this book. These "ground zero" notions are the cornerstones upon which successful teams of the future must be based. Second, Dr. Schulz reflects upon family issues which are relevant to teams of the present and the future but which are not addressed in the book. Finally, Dr. Fischer dreams a bit to project a few challenges that interdisciplinary teams of tomorrow will face.

RESONATING THEMES

The reader of this book has heard in the voices of all contributors a common plea: *Communicate!* This cry has been evident in chapter authors' presentations of discipline roles, in parents' questions, and in editorial responses. What can we do to communicate better?

We propose that an understanding of the communication process might help. Any basic communication course would describe this process as a transfer of information involving parties who serve both as senders and as receivers. Successful communication is largely dependent on active participation in these roles (Webster, 1977).

As senders, team members elect active participation when they carefully consider the abilities and needs of their communicative partners. That is, active senders form and deliver messages in ways that create the greatest probability of success. They don't assume that partners share their perspectives or are familiar with their terminology. Furthermore, they work hard to send messages that invite responses. Finally, active senders critically observe their partners. This allows for recognition and repair of communicative failures.

Active receivers listen with inquiring attitudes (Webster, 1977). This involves delaying judgment long enough to understand what another person thinks or feels. An active receiver also formulates and tests hypotheses which can provide windows to levels of meaning not apparent from a sender's literal message alone. For example, in a scenario in which team member "A" appears to ignore team member "B's" suggestions, team member "B" might state a hypothesis by saying, "This probably isn't the best time to talk." Team member "A's" response to this comment may provide insight that would otherwise be unavailable.

What else can be said about communicators who are active in their roles as senders and receivers? Three things come to mind. First, they communicate frequently. Nothing interrupts the team process more than the actual or perceived lack of communication. This book has provided numerous examples of how team members can communicate (e.g., face-to-face, in writing, electronically). We propose that all means of communication can be viable and that more is better than less when it comes to team communication. Second, active communicators are honest, yet sensitive. Team members (including family members) are entitled to each others' honest opinions. This doesn't mean that honesty can't be tempered with sensitivity. Most team members with any experience have observed good and bad examples of honesty and sensitivity; the Golden Rule probably provides the best guide. Finally, communicators who are active are not afraid of silence. Although silence during communication between team members can be intimidating, it can also provide opportunities for processing information and coping with emotions.

The second major theme of this book has been family-centeredness. Regardless of the team model selected, it is clearly apparent that teams of the future must be responsive to the needs and voices of families. For many team members this may mean rethinking what we've been taught. Some ancient adages come to mind: the child should not be considered separately from the family, the family knows the child better than the team member who is a discipline representative, and the family's priorities may be inconsistent with "best practice" from the perspective of professionals. Obviously, this list could continue.

Finally, we see empowerment as the key to family-centered teams of the future. Empowering families is critical to optimal outcomes for children with disabilities. How does this happen? We believe that families are empowered when professionals embrace and value the contributions of family members. It has been our observation that this occurs when there is an atmosphere of trust and mutual respect.

FAMILY ISSUES

Although a number of family issues have been addressed by the professionals in their chapters and by the parents' questions and comments, there are several issues that have not surfaced in either sector. The two that are most prominent by their omission are planning for the life span of the individual with a disability and preparing that individual for the role of self-advocacy.

As noted in Chapter 2, of the more than 500 responses to *The Bridging the Family-Professional Gap Family Member Survey*, there were very few family members with disabilities from age twenty to forty-one reported, and none beyond that age. This phenomenon raises several questions: Are parents of older individuals with disabilities more satisfied with the services they are receiving than are those of younger individuals? Are the problems encountered with younger children more challenging than those encountered with older individuals? Are parents of older individuals tired? Have they given up?

From reading this book one might conclude that the entire focus for individuals with disabilities begins at birth and ends with the completion of school. If we think of our children who do not have disabilities, we realize that this is the beginning–the preparation for life. The same concept applies to our children who have disabilities. There are many years beyond school, years full of challenges and opportunities.

Our family, like families represented in the survey, experienced many anxieties, frustrations, and uncertainties when Billy was a child. And yet, our most painful years have followed his graduation from high school. He was not prepared for living and working in the adult mainstream, nor were we prepared for the lack of information and services available to him and to us.

The transition component of IDEA has spawned many excellent programs and has created awareness in many communities of the needs and capabilities of young people who have disabilities. Such programs rely on teams composed of citizens in the community, service organizations, school personnel, and families of students with disabilities.

Some of our students with disabilities are progressing to postsecondary experiences and acquiring more advanced skills. I have always been puzzled by the idea that students with disabilities require less advanced training than other students. As parents and professionals, we need to promote the concept of adult education, which should be available to individuals covering the full range of disability.

In pursuing preparation for adult living in the mainstream, we should be concerned about issues of sexuality, options for independent living, more varied choices for work, and considerations of marriage and parenthood. Although many of us are concerned about the future of our children, in many cases we are not planning for it.

The ultimate goal for our children who have disabilities is for them to become advocates for their own rights and choices. One respondent in the survey stated that "family members are valuable members of the team, but we must also allow individuals who have disabilities to speak out and teach."

In recent years, we have seen groups of adults with disabilities advocating for their rights to public transportation, for access to buildings and facilities, and for political recognition. A dramatic event occurred a few years ago when students at Gallaudet College (for students who are hearing impaired) demanded, and obtained, a president who is hearing impaired. While this may not be the best criterion for an administrator, it was a prime example of self-advocacy.

Self-advocacy, like communication, begins early. In the home it begins with making choices of food and clothing, and being allowed the dignity of responsibility. Teachers of children who have severe disabilities can be observed offering pictures and encouraging their students to point to choices of activities, playmates, and reinforcers.

Early in my teaching career I attended a team meeting (then referred to as "staffing") concerning a student who had severe behavior and emotional problems. We were especially pleased to have a psychiatrist in attendance, and were amazed when he asked "Where is Mike?" We replied that he was on the playground with an attendant. I will never forget the psychiatrist's question: "If we were talking about you, would you want to be in here or out there?"

IDEA offers the opportunity for self-advocacy in suggesting that students participate as team members at the IEP meeting. When this is possible and practical, it has been found that the level of the meeting is more professional and that the goals and objectives are more relevant to the needs of the student.

The ability and desire to become an advocate develop from self-acceptance and the confidence gained with the acquisition of appropriate social, academic, emotional, and vocational skills. This challenging, on-going task requires the collaboration of everyone involved in planning for the individual with a disability.

The pay off is hearing Billy say, "I got a good life."

CHALLENGES FOR THE FUTURE

A recurrent theme throughout this book has been the need for, and sometimes difficulty with, communication: communication among team members and communication between professional teams and families. The ability to communicate will likely define the effectiveness of teams functioning in the future just as it does today. As we move more rapidly into the information age, advances in telecommunications will provide teams with new and increasingly more sophisticated challenges to their ability to communicate. Let us look briefly at how teams and families of the future might meet some of these challenges.

In Chapter 3, Dr. Eig, a pediatrician, laments his inability to participate in team meetings. He indicates that teams typically meet in schools or centers while he must remain in his office and hospital. In the future Dr. Eig or the team neurologist, ENT, orthopedic surgeon, and other professionals will be able to participate in team meetings via two-way interactive video-conferencing. Without leaving his office, the physician will be able to see, hear and respond to interactions among team members and families meeting at the local elementary school. If the physician or other team members cannot participate, even using video-conferencing, they will be able to review a video of the conference from their computer and make comments that can be watched later by other team members.

The impact of advances in telecommunication has the potential to affect every aspect of the team's interactions. Currently, professionals and family members try desperately to describe behaviors that each of them has observed in a child. If the old adage that a picture is worth a thousand words is true, how much would a video example be worth? In team meetings of the future all members, including the parents, will be able to show video examples of behaviors they have observed, therapy techniques, evaluation results, etc. Members who participate from remote locations using teleconferencing will likewise be able to see and show video examples.

In reviewing the responses of parents to our survey questions, it was clear that many parents who work outside the home felt frustration at not being able to observe or participate in their child's therapy sessions. Mothers and fathers who were not able to attend speech-language therapy, for example, indicated difficulty reinforcing behaviors at home that they had never seen modeled by the clinician. In the future, parents will be able to spend their lunch hours watching their child participating in speech, occupational and physical therapy, engaged in educational programs, or simply having fun on the playground. Further, they will be able to ask questions of teachers and therapists and receive immediate feedback.

Another area in which the future will improve communication is in the ability to obtain current information about specific disabilities. Several parents indicated their frustration in working with professionals who have had little experience with children who exhibit the same disability as their child. Especially for those professionals working in rural settings, the ability to collaborate with other professionals and learn more about a specific disability may be limited. In the future, professionals will have immediate access to the world's experts on any specific disability. This will include comprehensive web pages, video lectures, and examples of therapy and video-conferencing with colleagues around the world.

While this discussion has been limited to changes in the area of communication, it should be noted that advances in biomedical technology will likewise have a significant impact on individuals with disabilities and thus on families and teams. Every day the news is filled with reports of breakthroughs in genetic engineering, prenatal diagnosis and treatment, and advances in perinatal care. As these advances are applied to various disabilities, we can expect to see a clear shift from secondary and tertiary prevention (the therapy we currently provide) to primary prevention that will decrease or eliminate the incidence and severity of disabilities.

So, what will the challenges be for teams of the future? Team members, including families, will be challenged to become informed about new technologies, to acquire the skills to use them appropriately, and to apply such knowledge and ability to improve the quality of life for children and adults who have disabilities.

REFERENCES

Webster, E.J. (1977). *Counseling with parents of handicapped children: Guidelines for improving communication.* New York: Grune and Stratton.

EPILOGUE

In a book written in 1980, entitled *The Unexpected Minority* (Harcourt Brace Jonavovich), Gliedman and Roth described what a traveler from an advanced industrial society that respected the needs and the humanity of people with disabilities would expect to find on a visit to the United States. They compared this expectation with what the traveler would actually find: vast numbers of institutions where men, women, and children were left in solitude; work practices that systematically discriminated against disabled workers; a market structure in which information, innovation, and funds for capitalization of new ventures for individuals with disabilities are difficult to obtain; a neglect of the needs of the disabled in our man-made environments; the disabled individual portrayed as a child in our media; and disabled individuals as politically weak members of our society.

We would like to invite that traveler to return to the United States in 2025 and to find a society that, beginning with individuals at or before birth, accommodates persons with disabilities as it accommodates all people. Such accommodation would include full knowledge by all people of the needs, abilities, and potential of persons with disabilities. It would acknowledge the contributions that persons with disabilities can make to society in terms of business, politics, the arts, education, and family life. The traveler would see our society, including persons with disabilities, working together to create options and possibilities for all people.

Appendix 1

BRIDGING THE FAMILY-PROFESSIONAL GAP
FAMILY MEMBER SURVEY

A.   Please tell us about yourself:

1.   What is your relationship to your family member with a disability?
     _____mother   _____father   _____sister/brother
     _____grandparent   _____aunt/uncle   _____cousin
     _____other (please specify): _____

2.   Are you the primary caregiver for your family member with a disability?
     _____Yes   _____No

3.   If you answered "no" above, who is the primary caregiver?_____

4.   What is the occupation of the primary caregiver? _____

5.   What is the highest level of education the caregiver completed?
     _____elementary school   _____some trade/technical school
     _____middle school   _____trade/technical school
     _____some high school   _____college
     _____some college   _____Master's, Ph.D., M.D., etc.

6.   Which of the following ethnic classifications best describes your family?
     _____African-American _____Asian or Pacific Islander
     _____Caucasian   _____Hispanic   _____Native American
     _____Other (please specify):_____

7.   In which U.S. state do you live? _____

8.   Which of the following best describes your family?
     _____two-parent family _____single-parent family _____blended family

B.   Please tell us about your family member with a disability:

1.   What is the sex of your family member with a disability?
_____Female   _____Male

2.   What is the age (in years) of your family member? _____

3.   Please indicate below whether your family member with a disability is:
_____adopted   _____foster   _____neither of these

4.   Does your family member with a disability live at home?
_____Yes
_____No (Please specify where he/she lives): _____

5.   How many brothers and sisters does your family member have? _____

6.   In regard to birth order, what is your family member's position in the family?
_____only child
_____oldest child
_____middle child (or one of the middle children)
_____youngest child

7.   What is the nature of your family member's disability?
_____autism   _____orthopedic impairment
_____emotional/behavioral impairment   _____speech and/or language
                                           impairment
_____hearing impairment   _____visual impairment
_____learning disability   _____other
                                   (specify): _____

8.   How would you describe the severity of your family member's disability?
_____mild   _____moderate _____severe   _____profound

9.   How old (in years) was your family member when you first suspected that he/she had a problem? _____

10.   How old (in years) was your family member when the initial diagnosis was made by a professional? _____

11.   Who made the initial diagnosis? (Check one)
___audiologist   ___nurse   ___physician   ___speech-language
                                                     pathologist
___counselor   ___nutritionist ___psychologist ___ENT
                                                     (ear/nose/throat
                                                     physician)

___dentist   ___occupational ___social worker ___yourself
therapist
___neurologist ___physical   ___special educator ___other
therapist   (specify)_____

12. Which of the following professionals have been involved in planning or delivery of services to your family member?
___audiologist   ___nurse   ___physician   ___speech-language
pathologist
___counselor   ___nutritionist ___psychologist ___ENT
(ear/nose/throat
physician)
___dentist   ___occupational ___social worker ___other
therapist   (specify)_____
___neurologist ___physical therapist   ___special educator

13. Which of the following professionals have been the *primary providers* of services to your family member? (Check all that apply)
___audiologist   ___nurse   ___physician   ___speech-language
pathologist
___counselor   ___nutritionist ___psychologist ___ENT
(ear/nose/throat
physician)
___dentist   ___occupational ___social worker ___other
therapist   (specify)_____
___neurologist ___physical therapist   ___special educator

14. A *team* is a group of professional who work together to make decisions and carry out treatment for individuals with disabilities. Which of the following statements best describe the type of services provided to your family member?
_____My family member is served by individual professionals.
_____My family member is served by a team of professionals.

15. Is your family member with a disability currently enrolled in an educational program?
_____Yes   _____No

16. What is the highest level of education completed by your family member?
_____day care   _____high school
_____preschool   _____college
_____kindergarten   _____trade/technical school
_____elementary school   _____other
_____middle school   (please specify):_____

17.   How many years of special services has your family member received?
        _____

18.   If your family member with a disability is not in school, what is he/she
        doing now? _____

19.   If your family member is employed, which of the following best describes
        his/her type of employment?
        _____sheltered employment   _____competitive employment
        _____supportive employment   _____other
                                                 (please specify)_____

20.   How long have you lived in your community?
        _____

21.   Were needed services available in your community?
        _____Yes   _____No

22.   Was it necessary to relocate your family in order to obtain needed services?
        _____Yes   _____No

23.   Which best describes the type of community in which you live?
        _____suburban
        _____large city/urban area (more than 100,000 people)
        _____small city (25,000-100,000 people)
        _____rural

In answering questions 24-27, please rank each item by order of importance, with 1
being most important*:

24.   How did you feel when you were first told about your family member's
        disability?* (Please rank)
        _____angry   _____relieved
        _____confused   _____resentful
        _____guilty   _____other (please specify):_____
        _____numb

25.   What issues most concerned you about your family member's disability?*
        (Please rank)
        _____where to get help
        _____what to tell people
        _____what to expect in the future
        _____other(please specify):_____

26.   Which of the following resources have been of the greatest help to you?* (Please rank)

      _____professionals

      _____families of individuals with disabilities

      _____family support groups

      _____immediate and extended family

      _____other (please specify):_____

27.   How do you feel about your family member's disability now?* (Please rank)

      _____angry   _____relieved

      _____confused   _____resentful

      _____guilty   _____other (please specify):_____

      _____numb

C.   Please give us your comments to pass on to professionals:

1.   If you could raise any questions of team members, what would you ask and to whom would address your question?

2.   What advice would you give to professionals?

3.   If you could start over, what services would you seek?

4.   What aspect of your family member's disability has been most difficult for you to deal with?

5.   Are there other issues that you would like to raise relative to your past and present experiences working with professionals who serve the special needs of your family?

D.   Please tell us about your interactions with professionals:

1.   Professionals have a good understanding of the nature of my family member's disability.

    Strongly Agree.....Agree.....Disagree.....Strongly Disagree.....Does Not Apply

2. I understand my family member's disability.
   Strongly Agree.....Agree.....Disagree.....Strongly Disagree.....Does Not Apply

3. The program my family member is in has helped me understand his/her problem better.
   Strongly Agree.....Agree.....Disagree.....Strongly Disagree.....Does Not Apply

4. Professionals address my questions and concerns in a straightforward manner.
   Strongly Agree.....Agree.....Disagree.....Strongly Disagree.....Does Not Apply

5. Technical terms used by professionals are explained to me.
   Strongly Agree.....Agree.....Disagree.....Strongly Disagree.....Does Not Apply

6. The information I received about my family member's disability was presented in terms I could easily understand.
   Strongly Agree.....Agree.....Disagree.....Strongly Disagree.....Does Not Apply

7. I was given adequate information about my family member's disability.
   Strongly Agree.....Agree.....Disagree.....Strongly Disagree.....Does Not Apply

8. Professionals asked for my opinions and suggestions concerning my family member's disability, treatment and education.
   Strongly Agree.....Agree.....Disagree.....Strongly Disagree.....Does Not Apply

9. Professionals fully informed me about my family member's disability, current level of functioning and outlook for future functioning.
   Strongly Agree.....Agree.....Disagree.....Strongly Disagree.....Does Not Apply

10. The responsibilities of each team member were fully explained to me.
    Strongly Agree.....Agree.....Disagree.....Strongly Disagree.....Does Not Apply

11. It was easy to get help for my family member.
    Strongly Agree.....Agree.....Disagree.....Strongly Disagree.....Does Not Apply

12. Professionals treated my family with compassion.
    Strongly Agree.....Agree.....Disagree.....Strongly Disagree.....Does Not Apply

13. Professionals were honest and sincere.
    Strongly Agree.....Agree.....Disagree.....Strongly Disagree.....Does Not Apply

14. Professionals viewed my family in a positive light.
    Strongly Agree.....Agree.....Disagree.....Strongly Disagree.....Does Not Apply

15. Professionals valued my family's knowledge, opinions and observations.
    Strongly Agree.....Agree.....Disagree.....Strongly Disagree.....Does Not Apply

16. Professionals' advice was worth following.
Strongly Agree.....Agree.....Disagree.....Strongly Disagree.....Does Not Apply

17. I was satisfied with the intervention plan.
Strongly Agree.....Agree.....Disagree.....Strongly Disagree.....Does Not Apply

18. The program my family member is in seems to be helping him/her.
Strongly Agree.....Agree.....Disagree.....Strongly Disagree.....Does Not Apply

19. Family members had regular contact with professionals.
Strongly Agree.....Agree.....Disagree.....Strongly Disagree.....Does Not Apply

20. Professionals focused on understanding the needs and priorities of my family.
Strongly Agree.....Agree.....Disagree.....Strongly Disagree.....Does Not Apply

21. The needs and priorities of my family set the direction for treatment.
Strongly Agree.....Agree.....Disagree.....Strongly Disagree.....Does Not Apply

22. Professionals provided support by helping my family make its own decisions about needed services and intervention goals.
Strongly Agree.....Agree.....Disagree.....Strongly Disagree.....Does Not Apply

23. Professionals helped me learn new skills to get resources to meet my needs.
Strongly Agree.....Agree.....Disagree.....Strongly Disagree.....Does Not Apply

24. The team helped me plan for my child's transition from school to work.
Strongly Agree.....Agree.....Disagree.....Strongly Disagree.....Does Not Apply

25. All the professionals on the team were equally helpful to me.
Strongly Agree.....Agree.....Disagree.....Strongly Disagree.....Does Not Apply

26. My family was fully included in assessing our family member's problem, making decisions about needed services and carrying out the treatment plan.
Strongly Agree.....Agree.....Disagree.....Strongly Disagree.....Does Not Apply

Your return of this survey will indicate your informed consent and willingness to participate in the book project.
May we use your comments *anonymously* in the book?

_____ Yes, you may use my comments in the book. I understand they will be anonymous.

_____ No, I do not wish you to use my comments.

If you answered "Yes" above, please complete the section below. By doing so, you will receive information on the book.

If you would like, please provide the following information:
Name _____
Address _____
City _____ State _____ Zip Code _____
Electronic Mail Address _____
Thank you for taking the time to provide us with this important information.

AUTHOR INDEX

SUBJECT INDEX

277